FROM CHAOS TO COERCION

FROM CHAOS TO COERCION

Detention and the Control of Tuberculosis

Richard Coker

St. Martin's Press
New York

ISBN 0-312-22250-5

Library of Congress Cataloging-in-Publication Data

Coker, Richard J., 1960-
    From chaos to coercion : detention and the control of tuberculosis
  / Richard J. Coker.
      p.   cm.
    Includes bibliographical references and index.
    ISBN 0-312-22250-5 (cloth)
      1. Tuberculosis—New York (State)—New York.   2. Patient
  compliance—New York (State)—New York.3. Detention of persons-
  -New York (State)—New York. I. Title.
      [DNLM: 1. Tuberculosis—prevention & control—United States.
  2. Health Policy—United States.3. Patient Compliance—United
  States. WF200 C682f 2000]
  RC309.N7C64   2000
  362.1'96995'009747—dc21
  DNLM/DLC
  for Library of Congress   99-30119
                                                                       CIP

Design by Acme Art, Inc.
Printed in the United States of America

First edition: February 2000
10 9 8 7 6 5 4 3 2 1

For Helen,
my wife and best friend,
and my sons, Joseph and Jack

*Homeless, friendless, dependant, dissipated
and vicious consumptives are likely to be most
dangerous to the community.*

*—Hermann Biggs,
New York City Health Department, 1903*

CONTENTS

LIST OF FIGURES

ABBREVIATIONS

ACET	Advisory Council for the Elimination of Tuberculosis
ADA	Americans with Disabilities Act
AFDC	Aid for Families with Dependent Children
AIDS	Acquired immunodeficiency syndrome
CDC	Centers for Disease Control and Prevention
CDSC	Centre for Disease Surveillance and Control
DOC	Department of Correction
DOT	Directly observed therapy
EIS	Epidemic Intelligence Service
HHC	Health and Hospitals Corporation
HiB	*Haemophilus influenzae* type B
HIV	Human immunodeficiency virus
HMO	Health maintenance organization
HRA	Human Resources Administration
HUD	Department of Housing and Urban Development
MDRTB	Multidrug-resistant tuberculosis
OMB	Office of Management and Budget
OSHA	Occupational Safety and Health Act
PHA	public health advisor
PRA	Personal Responsibility and Work Opportunity Reconciliation Act
RFLP	Restriction fragment length polymorphism
SRO	Single-room occupancy hotel
SSI	Supplemental Security Income
STP	Supervised treatment program
TANF	Temporary Assistance for Needy Families
WHO	World Health Organization

FOREWORD

Before I built a wall I'd ask to know
What I was walling in or walling out,
And to whom I was like to give offence.
Something there is that doesn't love a wall,
That wants it down . . .

[My neighbor] will not go beyond his father's saying,
And he likes having thought of it so well
He says again, "Good fences make good neighbours."

—Robert Frost, "Mending Wall," 1920

(a) The Surgeon General, with the approval of the Secretary, is authorized to make and enforce such regulations as in his judgment are necessary to prevent the introduction, transmission, or spread of communicable diseases from foreign countries into the States or possessions, or from one State or possession into any other State or possession. . . .

(b) Regulations prescribed under this section shall not provide for apprehension, detention, or conditional release of individuals except for the purpose of preventing the introduction, transmission, or spread of such communicable diseases as may be specified from time to time in Executive orders of the President upon the recommendation or the National Advisory Health Council and the Surgeon General. . . .

(d) Such regulations may provide that if upon examination any such individual is found to be infected, he may be detained for such time and in such manner as may be reasonably necessary.

—Section 361, U.S. Public Health Service Act (42 U.S.C. 264)

Robert Frost would rather not take the trouble to build a wall between an apple orchard and a pine forest, but his neighbor and his neighbor's father before him have always built them. So they keep building them, wearing their hands rough with the handling of heavy stones.

Congress believed the act of quarantining a person (as opposed to animals or articles in commerce) was so serious a matter that it limited the surgeon general to taking action only in accordance with executive orders issued by the president, a high threshold in American law. But once that threshold is crossed, the surgeon general can do anything he or she finds "reasonably necessary."

This is the delicate balance in American law between individual liberty and public good. It is generally believed that personal freedom should be unrestricted unless the collective safety or welfare of other people requires that it be limited. In those instances in which society concludes that freedom should be restricted, however, limitations are sometimes far-reaching.

(It is almost certainly coincidental but nonetheless illuminating that the quarantine statute just cited was passed by Congress in 1944, the same year that the Supreme Court affirmed the decision that it was permissible for U.S. citizens of Japanese ancestry to be forced to leave their homes and live in internment camps. This action, which has since been widely denounced and for which the Congress has voted reparations payments, was justified on the basis of the "pressing public necessity.")

Richard Coker has examined this balance in the United States and found it to be not always so delicate. All of us can agree that it is a good thing to immunize children, care for mentally ill persons, and control tuberculosis. But Coker's observations about the use of what he calls "coercion" to achieve these goals suggest more control and less liberty than is usually part of the American self-image. His comments about the role of cultural differences—both within the United States and between the United States and the United Kingdom—lead one to look beneath "commonsense" public health measures to a much more complex conundrum of how to treat illness and prevent the spread of disease.

Such questions about correlations between coercion and disease control are key to both public health and civil liberties. A policy that shoots in the dark until it hits its target is dangerous to all concerned; it may fail to protect the populace effectively while regimenting it unnecessarily. In most instances, employing mandatory measures before voluntary options have been attempted seems trigger-happy and reckless. Why impose quarantine on patients who simply need help finding a doctor? Why confine people if what they need is assistance in paying for medical care? Why coerce people to behave in a desired way before enlisting their agreement?

One answer suggested by Coker's analysis is that mandatory measures may be easier. In a society in which low-income individuals often have no doctors, medical care, or insurance, the creation of a system in which they can voluntarily perform like "model citizens" would be complicated. When homelessness, HIV/AIDS, substance abuse, and poverty are added to the problem, it is far easier to respond with a single-purpose, coercive intervention than to provide for these people's comprehensive care. The self-defeating nature of this targeted response is visible only when the next health problem appears.

Another answer suggested by Coker's work may be the ad hoc nature of American public policy. We Americans may preach aphorisms like "an ounce of prevention is worth a pound of cure," but we rarely practice them. Modern America is a society that quite literally lets bridges fall down before adopting a program of routine bridge maintenance. It is a society that let its public funding for immunizations decline until there was an outbreak, responded with millions of dollars all at once, and is now investigating into why those millions have not been well budgeted while once again cutting immunization programs. In such a system, all parties wait for crises that demand immediate action and generally are uninterested in prudent long-term planning. Just as Las Vegas is the glittering icon of the American dreams of chance and instant money, our preventive health programs often are the sobering example of our willful disbelief in epidemiology and investment. With such a national mind-set, policymakers often leave themselves only mandatory measures to deal with public risks.

None of this is to say that there are not instances in which mandates are not appropriate. Without much trouble, examples can be conjured up of Typhoid Marys and malicious spreaders of disease. But what Coker's study suggests and what we must believe to be true is that these situations are the exception, not the general rule. If that is the case, the reflexive choice of mandatory measures for response is a non sequitur.

It need not always be so. A recent example of a more successful American initiative is the reduction of mother-to-child transmission of human immunodeficiency virus (HIV). After the discovery that anti-viral drugs administered during pregnancy could significantly reduce the chance of the baby being infected, there were immediate discussions of mandatory programs. Some suggested mandatory testing of pregnant women; others, paradoxically, used these findings to propose mandatory testing of infants.

Rather than adopting either of these approaches, however, the Public Health Service recommended that all physicians offer testing to pregnant women and, if they were infected, offer these women treatment. The results have been dramatic. Pediatric infection rates have fallen steeply, and some public hospitals that serve large numbers of adults with acquired immunodeficiency syndrome (AIDS) have had no newborns with HIV in over a year.

Such success may not be readily generalizable to other populations and other diseases. Pregnant women in the United States are more often eligible for government-assisted healthcare than are nonpregnant women or all men, and the efforts to recruit women into comprehensive programs of prenatal care have been increased like no other area of primary care. Homeless men with tuberculosis have few programs for their care structured and financed so well.

But there is much to be learned from Coker's studies of coercion and this example of prevention of pediatric HIV. The tension between the public good and individual liberty may often be a false dichotomy. More often than not, good public health policy is good civil liberties policy. Health practitioners and lawmakers should note that mandatory measures are often unnecessary if the basic elements of voluntary response are made available to those who need them.

This is an important and hopeful lesson. Coker does a lucid and insightful analysis of a great deal of history and policy that is short-sighted, ineffective, unfair, and sad. But by laying this analysis out so clearly, he has shown us a possible way to a public health enlightenment, a rebirth in the political faith in an informed public. If such a way ultimately leads to a time in which we direct our efforts to effective measures rather than reactive ones, we will have made great progress. We can spend less time "walling in or walling out" and more time meeting the genuine needs of all members of our society.

Tim Westmoreland
Georgetown University Law Center, May 1999

PREFACE AND ACKNOWLEDGMENTS

The idea for this work came while I had the privilege of studying in the United States on a Harkness Fellowship. This is a remarkably generous program funded by The Commonwealth Fund of New York. Jack O'Sullivan, Pamela Gillies, and Mark Poznansky, all of whom had, a few years earlier, been Harkness fellows, suggested I apply. Their advice was excellent. Before leaving for the United States I had been contemplating the global increase in cases of tuberculosis, the threat of drug-resistant strains, the problems of noncompliant patients under my care, and in particular the case of one particular patient, Paul Mayho (of whom more in chapter one). The problem of tuberculosis control, it seemed to me, could be viewed as a medical problem, a social problem, or, more appropriately, a complex biosocial problem. Although the medical approach might be, in the short term, somewhat simpler, I felt it was only a Band-Aid; with this approach the problem still lay below the surface ready to reappear when the temporary covering (of medical support) was removed. The success of the New York response in turning the tide had received international recognition, and I was curious to find out what lay behind this success, why the tide had needed to be turned in the first place, and whether the lessons being drawn are transferable elsewhere. This book is the result of my research.

Many might take as unacceptable the views of an outsider (and a somewhat critical outsider at that). Yet I make no apologies for this, for if we are to learn from the lessons of New York, from both its successes and failures, then what happened must be opened up to analysis to those from a variety of perspectives, native and foreign. I have not intended, in this book, to deprecate the substantial achievements in tuberculosis control that have been made in New York over the past seven or eight years; I have attempted to appraise the approach taken, place it in context, and draw lessons that might be useful both in the United States and elsewhere. In particular, I have not attempted a detailed analysis of the response overall but focused on an illustrative aspect, that of detention of recalcitrant individuals. If we are to contemplate the adoption of similar approaches, as some in Europe are suggesting, for example, we must be aware of the cultural and social milieu in which the New York City epidemic flourished. Just as the HIV-infected person may serve, like the miner's canary, as an early warning system for tuberculosis, so too might New York serve as a warning system for the health consequences of social policies that neglect the most vulnerable. And, paradoxically, New York City's response might serve both as a beacon and warning light to those facing public health problems of their own.

This book would not have been possible without the enormous support from a large number of people. I am especially grateful to Professor Ronald Bayer, of Columbia University, who guided me, intellectually challenged and stimulated me, and offered great support throughout this venture; Dr. Paula Fujiwara, of the New York City Bureau of Tuberculosis Control, for the unfettered access she gave me to her staff and internal bureau documents and for explaining to me the workings of the public health program, both past and present; and Dr. John Porter, of The London School of Hygiene and Tropical Medicine, who, through some difficult times for me, unstintingly and gently encouraged me to further my research and complete it as a book. I am grateful also to Professor Tim Westmoreland, of Georgetown University, who over the years has given up his time unsparingly to describe the intricacies of the American political and legal processes, assisted me in formulating my interpretations of the politics of health in America, and helped me to clarify many of my ramblings and musings.

I am indebted to the many employees of the New York City Bureau of Tuberculosis Control, from both before 1993 and after, who gave up so much of their time, clarified my misunderstandings, and answered my unending questions so patiently. They include: Gail Cairns, Pat Carrusso, José Castro, Marie Dorsinville, Dr. Gabe Feldman, Dr. Thomas Frieden, Rose Gasner, Christina Larkin, Dr. Lilla Lyon, Dr. Sonal Munsiff, Laurie Nathan, and many more I have not listed. Several detained individuals offered me their insights and told me about their lives, and I thank them for their frankness and trust. I also thank the many patients who offered me their perspective while receiving directly observed therapy (DOT) and the public health advisors who showed me "their" system. Lawyers acting for both sides, the city and the detainees, were remarkably frank and open, and I owe them a debt of gratitude. I am also beholden to the many people who gave up their time willingly and allowed themselves to be interviewed and who requested anonymity. These requests have been honored.

Many physicians, from New York and beyond, helped clarify and refine my analysis. In particular I am grateful to Dr. Karen Brudney, Dr. Richard Chaisson, Dr. Eran Bellin, Dr. Wafaa El-Sadr, Dr. Paul Farmer, Dr. Mindy Fullilove, Dr. Barron Lerner, Dr. Ed Nardell, and Dr. Neil Schluger.

A special thank you must go to Dr. J. R. Willie Harris, of St. Mary's Hospital, who has been an inspirational support for many years. He, along with Dr. David Mitchell, encouraged me to develop my interest in tuberculosis further; I learned much from their teaching and integrity. Many of my colleagues at Imperial College, London, with whom I am affiliated academically, are also owed a debt of gratitude for their support.

Paul Mayho, with whom I spent many hours talking, forced me to contemplate the hardships we as doctors place upon our patients, the harm we can unwittingly do, and how much we often expect but how little we have to offer in return.

Thanks are also due to Professor James Morone, of Brown University, and Professor Amy Fairchild and Professor David Rosner, of Columbia University, for their insights, and contagious enthusiasm.

I owe a special debt of gratitude to Karen Davis, president of The Commonwealth Fund of New York, who, in addition to the Harkness Fellowship, provided me with additional support through a presidential grant to work on the manuscript of this book. The Jefferiss Trust also assisted me financially during the manuscript completion.

All of the people named above, and all those whom I have failed to name but have helped with this project, bear no responsibility for any factual errors, inconsistencies, or ill thought out arguments in this book.

I am grateful to my parents for all their support over the years. This book is dedicated to my wife and two sons. Helen has encouraged, cajoled, edited, and proofread all of my work. Her inspiration turned what was chaotic into something cogent. She, like my children, Joseph and Jack, has lived with my uncertainties and moods when troubles at work threatened to engulf me. Each and all of them have carried me through.

The author and publisher are grateful to the following institutions and people for permission to reproduce figures: American Society of Law, Medicine & Ethics, Karen Bonuck, and Peter Arno (figure 3.2), and the American Economic Association (figure 3.3).

FROM CHAOS TO COERCION

1

Introduction

Tuberculosis is a social disease, and presents problems that transcend the conventional medical approach. On the one hand, its understanding demands that the impact of social and economic factors on the individual be considered as much as the mechanisms by which tubercle bacilli cause damage to the human body. On the other hand, the disease modifies in a peculiar manner the emotional and intellectual climate of the societies that it attacks.

—René and Jean Dubos,
The White Plague: Tuberculosis, Man, and Society, 1952

The United States, and in particular New York City, witnessed an alarming increase in tuberculosis rates during the 1980s. Indeed, the epidemic of tuberculosis in New York was one of the more dramatic epidemics the West has endured in the last 30 years (and was closely allied to the human immunodeficiency virus [HIV] epidemic in that city) but has received surprisingly little attention outside of local news media and the specialist American medical literature. The epidemic was associated with an increase in incidence of multidrug-resistant tuberculosis (MDRTB), particularly in HIV-infected individuals. The percentage of cases resistant to at least one drug rose from 19 percent in 1987 to 28 percent in 1991, while rates of MDRTB rose from 6 percent to 14 percent, most of it "home-grown."[1] Nosocomial spread, or clustering related to spread within congregate settings such as hospitals, shelters for the homeless, and prisons, made a substantial contribution to the increase.[2] New York City responded with a range of initiatives including the widespread use of directly observed therapy (DOT) to improve both completion-of-treatment rates and treatment compliance. To underpin this strategy, coercive public health measures were introduced that gave the commissioner of health the authority to mandate DOT and, as a last resort, to detain individuals "where there is a substantial likelihood, based on such person's past or present behavior, that he or she can not be relied upon to participate in and/or to complete an appropriate prescribed course of medication for tuberculosis and/or, if necessary, to follow required contagion precautions for tuberculosis."[3]

This book uses the lens of tuberculosis, that "perfect expression of an imperfect civilisation," and the regulatory changes that ensued from New York City's contemporary tuberculosis epidemic, to examine the American response to those who pose a threat to others through their failure to conform. Their poor and inadequate compliance with treatment means they risk relapsing (or remaining persistently infectious) and, the worst scenario of all, transmitting drug-resistant strains of tuberculosis to others who then go on to develop disease. Because this still-stigmatized disease is transmitted in a casual fashion (mainly through coughing, unlike, for example, HIV), the tensions between the rights and responsibilities of many of the most marginalized individuals and societal obligations to its most vulnerable are thrown into stark relief. In addition, therefore, to examining the response to some of society's most chaotic individuals (who have, we must remember, committed no crime), I also reflect upon whether society should be held at least in part responsible for the antisocial and chaotic behavior of some of its members. If, as I suggest, this is the case, then the moral issues regarding detention of those who are not infectious but persist in failing to comply with treatment are complex. Only by examining the causes of the tuberculosis epidemic that swept through New York City in the late 1980s and early 1990s, the context in which the seeds of both recalcitrance and tuberculosis were sown, *and* the response to the epidemic can we hope to draw lessons. Too simplistic an analysis, by looking only at the response, threatens to provide only simplistic answers.

What prompted me to write this book? London, where I work as a consultant physician, has for several years seen an increase in tuberculosis rates. All of us who look after patients with tuberculosis have come across "difficult" patients, those who, for whatever reason, find it difficult or are unwilling to comply with their treatment. By and large, through a variety of means (cajoling, bribing with meals and snacks, encouraging through frequent telephone contact, improving housing or other social hurdles, etc.), most complete their treatment. But a few are "lost," and often what happens to them is unclear. Although I had been concerned about these patients and the public health implications, they had been so few in number, and there were so many other pressing problems, not least the social problems of the patients who continued to come to the clinic, that my attention was not held by these "recalcitrant" individuals. But then, on Thursday August 10, 1995, I met one particular patient, Paul Mayho, who caused me to reflect a little more.

Paul is a bright, articulate gay man. He had developed acquired immunodeficiency syndrome (AIDS) about 18 months before I met him and received his care at another London teaching hospital. He had recently been admitted there complaining of diarrhea. While an inpatient he had shared a ward with several other patients, all of whom were also HIV seropositive. Toward the end of his stay a new patient arrived, somebody who would change all their lives forever. This new patient had been admitted for investigation and treatment of a respiratory illness. His illness, it later transpired, was multidrug-resistant tuberculosis, from which he died. Shortly thereafter many of the patients sharing the same ward area became ill. One by one each patient was diagnosed with MDRTB.[4] And one by one they died. This strain of disease threatened to be as untreatable as that signalled by Keats's first spots of blood on his handkerchief, his "death warrant."

Paul, when he came to see me, was frightened. He had been started on a range of different, unpleasant drugs and was suffering from several side effects, was severely immunocompromised, and, even without the development of tuberculosis, faced a grim, short future. Like those in the preantibiotic era, ahead of him lay the possibility of an increasing struggle for breath, the possibility of hemorrhage into his lungs, and an inexorable wasting away. He had already started to lose weight and, most worryingly, had developed a cough. The future did not portend well. And he was infectious. Examination of his stained sputum showed hundreds of bright-red tubercle bacilli.

Paul spent the next three months isolated in a small room in the hospital. The psychological trauma was perhaps even greater than the physical.[5] At the time of his admission I had estimated, and told him, he might live six more months. As the days spread to weeks he could see what little life remained to him slipping away. Many of his friends and work colleagues were HIV seropositive. His contact with the outside world was restricted to the few visitors he was allowed and his television and radio. His room at St. Mary's Hospital still bares the marks etched on the wall, each mark representing a day. There are nearly one hundred.

What struck me most about Paul, and is recorded in his published diaries, was his automatic, unqualified acceptance of his social responsibility.[6] His anger arose from the injustice of having perhaps his last months of life taken from him "through no fault of his own." Yet he recognized his wider social responsibilities, his duty to protect the wider public from "his" tuberculosis.

Remarkably Paul is, four years later, well and perhaps fitter than he has been in years. The advent of effective anti-HIV treatment, and his persistence in adhering for over two years with his antituberculosis treatment (including thrice-weekly intramuscular injections for a substantial part of that) has meant that his life has been resurrected. He is again back at work and cured of his tuberculosis.

What would we have done if Paul had refused to be isolated, if he had refused all treatment, or if he had wanted to spend what little time appeared to be left to him at liberty in the city? And what would we have done if, after six months of treatment, by which time he had become noninfectious, he had had enough of doctors, hospitals, and drugs? In Britain the public health legislation is unclear regarding the powers at our disposal.[7] But even if they were clear, and detention for noncompliant noninfectious individuals could be authorized, would we have been morally justified in using these powers? New York faced these questions, through force of circumstance, in the early 1990s.

Like Paul Mayho, John Keats, the Brontë sisters, Chekhov, George Orwell, and millions of others unknown have had tuberculosis. They, unlike Paul but like millions each year even now, died from their disease. Yet what separates Keats and his fellow mortal consumptives from Paul and his contemporaries is that tuberculosis need no longer be a "death warrant." Effective treatment is available today and has been so for several decades. Yet today tuberculosis kills more people than any other infectious disease. The World Health Organization (WHO) estimates that perhaps a third of the world's population harbor the bacterium, and are infected with *M. tuberculosis,* and nearly 8 million develop disease each year. Of those 8 million, 3 million die, including 100,000 children. How is it that this medical condition can overwhelm our medical knowledge and medical approaches? Because tuberculosis is, as René and Jean Dubos recognized nearly 50 years ago, first and foremost a social condition. And it is for this reason that it continues to defy us—and enthral us.

Tuberculosis has been afflicting mankind for as long as humans have walked the earth. It is a disease steeped in history and its synonyms (consumption, phthisis, the king's evil, white death) conjure up romantic images of pale, wraith-like artists lying prostrate coughing blood, suffering lingering deaths. Through the eighteenth, nineteenth, and early twentieth centuries tuberculosis transformed the lives of its victims and their families, and influenced literature, art, music, and society. Those who succumbed to the disease form a veritable who's who of the artistic world (e.g., Samuel Johnson, Sir Walter Scott, Frederic Chopin, Elizabeth Barrett Browning, Anthony Trollope, Fyodor Dostoevsky, Anton Chekhov, and many others). And they, or their friends, recorded the effects of the disease so that our perceptions continue, to this day, to be infused with romantic notions. As Susan Sontag suggested in her book *Illness as Metaphor,* in the nineteenth century "TB was understood, like insanity, to be a kind of one-sidedness: a failure of will or an overintensity. However much the disease was dreaded, TB always had pathos. Like the mental patient today, the tubercular was considered to be someone quintessentially vulnerable, and full of self-destructive whim" and, in support of the notion that those with artistic leanings were particularly susceptible she noted that "TB was thought to come from too much passion, afflicting the reckless and sensual."[8]

But the disease was not limited to those with an artistic temperament; it was simply that the disease was endemic, that it was one of the greatest causes of death and disease in the West, and it defined much artistic work during this period. The poor were carried off by it in their millions. Thomas Dormandy, in his recent history of tuberculosis has suggested that, "With poverty, malnutrition, overcrowding, vice, crime, and moral degradation it became not just a cause or consequence but part of the landscape of the Industrial Revolution."[9] As factories went up from the 1800s and urban poverty grew, tuberculosis rates soared among the poor. As this popular awareness of the class associations of the disease became clearer (and the discovery that it was a bacterial infection) tuberculosis started to lose its romantic attachments. Charles Dickens' "dread disease" continues to capture the public imagination, provoking fear, a fear that not only one might catch the disease but also, perhaps subliminally, that one might become infected with the same "flaws"—alcoholism, drug-dependency, poverty—that those with the disease seem predisposed to.

COMPLIANCE, ADHERENCE, CONCORDANCE, AND DOT

There has been, over the past few years, a debate in health policy circles about the terminology regarding treatment. Many suggest, rightly, that the term "compliance" in regard to treatment describes, in addition to patients taking their prescribed treatment, a power relationship between the doctor and patient; the patient "follows doctor's orders," the patient is passive and the doctor paternalistic. As a consequence some have suggested that the terms "adherence" or "concordance" should be used instead.[10] Both these terms, it has been argued, lend greater authority to patient autonomy. They suggest that the doctor-patient relationship is more of an equal partnership rather than one of dominator and supplicant. The patient's agenda is given greater respect with these terms. While both terms suggest that the clinical encounter between patient and doctor is equal, they also indicate that both have different roles to play. The patient's task is voluntary; she has the opportunity to negotiate depending on her health beliefs. I have, however, decided not to use these terms in this book because the power play between doctors and patients, when it comes to communicable diseases such as tuberculosis, is by its nature very different than for most other medical conditions. The threat to others is hardly an issue when a doctor is prescribing antihypertensives or anti-inflammatory drugs. Yet when it comes to the treatment of tuberculosis, public health concerns are always asserting a force on the doctor-patient relationship, threatening to make the relationship unequal. For this reason the term "compliance" has been used throughout this book.

In chapter 4 I describe how Christopher Foreman of The Brookings Institution suggests that health reporters are drawn to four kinds of stories: fire alarms, controversies, human interest, and breakthroughs.[11] While much of the early part of this book describes how the first three of these stories caught the public imagination and defined the response, it is perhaps the last that is influencing global policy on tuberculosis control to the greatest extent. A brief diversion is, therefore, warranted.

Directly observed therapy was taken up by the WHO recently as the "breakthrough" in tuberculosis control, a position that can be ascribed in large part to the achievements in bringing the New York City epidemic under control (and also two other American examples, Baltimore and Tarrant County, Texas).[12] DOT, a system that requires a health worker to watch as a patient takes his mediation, is being aggressively pursued by the WHO and is now the standard of care in treatment in the United States.[13]

In order to enhance compliance through DOT, legal leverage was viewed as necessary in New York. DOT was at the heart of the response, and its expansion, I suggest, killed several birds with one stone. First it ensured compliance with treatment; second (as a consequence of the former) it reduced the development of drug resistance; third it increased public health authority over patients, enabling them to be "policed"; and finally it increased public health officials' credibility before clinicians treating recalcitrant tuberculosis patients.

Although there were only a few DOT enthusiasts in the United States, notably in Denver and Baltimore, before the 1990s, others lent their support when the scale of the potential threat and its associated cost implications from multidrug-resistant strains became clear.[14] Emblematic of this shift was the attention given to the widely referenced title of a 1993 *New England Journal* Sounding Board article, "Directly Observed Treatment Of Tuberculosis: We Can't Afford Not to Try It," written by three Denver-based experts advancing the notion of universal DOT.[15] The benefits of the system hinged on the enhancement of treatment compliance, the consequent low relapse rate and low rates of acquired drug resistance, and the cost benefits when compared to standard self-administered treatment.[16]

Often policymakers forget that the ultimate goal of tuberculosis programs is not to make as many patients as possible complete therapy but to reduce the incidence of tuberculosis, including drug-resistant tuberculosis, in a community. So one must ask, have alternative approaches to preventing relapse and the subsequent development of drug resistance been considered adequately, and if not, why not? And is DOT morally justifiable and culturally acceptable?

Drug resistance occurs when only one drug is taken, which gives organisms already resistant to this drug a selective advantage. When a further drug is added, a few organisms that have spontaneously mutated gain a further selective advantage. Drug-resistant and then multidrug-resistant strains ensue. Fixed-dose combinations of antituberculosis drugs combine two or more drugs, making it impossible for patients to receive monotherapy. These combinations have been used extensively in some countries, such as Brazil, Spain, and the United Kingdom. Even where control programs are poorly administered or resourced, drug-resistant tuberculosis is an infrequent problem where fixed-dose drug combinations are widely used.[17] In the United Kingdom, for example, where treatment compliance in many parts of the country may be inadequately monitored and there are no data on completion-of-treatment rates, it has been estimated that between 73 to 79 percent of rifampin, the most potent antituberculosis drug available, is sold as a constituent in fixed combinations. Although tuberculosis rates are climbing, the incidence of drug resistance and multidrug resistance is very low.[18] Similar situations are found in Brazil and Spain. By comparison, in the United States, with higher rates of drug resistance, less than 20 percent of rifampin is sold in such formulations,[19] and in many other countries with substantial MDRTB rates fixed-dose drug combinations are rarely used. But neither the United States nor the WHO is an enthusiastic supporter of adopting more widespread use of this approach, and there is little evidence of support for future research to evaluate its potential benefit. All eggs are in the DOT basket.

DOT (or supervised therapy, as it was earlier called) has a lengthy history of enhancing tuberculosis treatment.[20] It has shown advantages over standard unsupervised self-administered treatment, but recent research findings question the need for universal DOT in practical terms. For example, in some studies, under programs with low completion-of-treatment rates DOT has a marked impact; but where completion-of-treatment rates are already over 90 percent, a switch to universal DOT is probably unnecessary and provides little additional benefit.[21] Between 1990, when only about 60 percent of patients were completing treatment in New York City, and 1994, when nearly 90 percent were, the DOT program was expanded, but never more than 50 percent of patients have been enrolled. Factors other than DOT clearly have contributed substantially to the improvement in rates of treatment completion; such factors include departmental leadership, the commitment and vigor of caregivers, improved surveillance, and heightened citywide awareness of the problem. At other sites the impact of DOT has been questioned. In South Africa, for example, a trial comparing DOT and self-supervised treatment showed little difference in outcome between the two groups.[22] In Botswana another recent study showed that, despite the implementation of a DOT-based program, tuberculosis control is failing.[23] So DOT may not necessarily be the answer, or even part of the answer.[24] Yet DOT remains the official "gold standard," and most experts suggest that it should be one of *the* components to an effective program. Why is this?

National comparisons, and even intranational comparisons, suggest fixed-dose combination treatment offers benefits over standard unsupervised treatment.[25] There appears to be little difference in terms of relapse rates or drug-resistance development when fixed-dose drug combinations are compared with supervised treatment.[26] But even though three trials comparing combined preparations with standardized treatment lend weight to the use of fixed-dose combinations (both because marginally more rapid sputum clearance can be achieved and no difference in rates of acquired drug resistance occurred), support in the United States and at the WHO is muted.[27] This may be, in part, because the U.S. trial had an insufficient number of patients who failed treatment to establish the value, or lack thereof, of combined preparations. (Somewhat ironically, this was the only trial that compared fixed combinations with self-administered treatment.) In the other two trials treatment was supervised.[28] Only one trial showed a significant difference in relapse rates (p = 0.04), which were slightly higher in the fixed-formulation group, but in no trials was drug resistance increased.[29] All in all, therefore, the case for DOT above self-administered fixed-dose drug combinations has not been proven.

What about the cost effectiveness of different approaches? Very little research has been conducted to evaluate the cost benefit of fixed-dose combination treatment. Merrick Zwarenstein and his colleagues from the Medical Research Council, Tygerberg, South Africa, recently published a study that showed no advantage over using DOT, and estimated that DOT cost three times more than self-supervised treatment.[30] Only one paper, from Richard Chaisson's group in Baltimore, has compared self-administration, DOT, and fixed-dose treatment.

These researchers showed that both DOT and fixed-combination treatment were more cost effective than unsupervised treatment in the Baltimore setting.[31] They concluded that there was little difference between the two approaches (fixed dose and DOT) in terms of cost effectiveness. Further cost-benefit analysis is obviously warranted for other nonurban areas and for other countries, both developing and in the West. Assessing the cost of treating tuberculosis with fixed-dose combinations is clearly more complex than a simple calculation of the cost of the different drug formulations. The human and economic costs of drug resistance arising from inappropriate use of single-formulation drugs and of the implementation of and ongoing costs of DOT should be weighed against the costs of fixed-drug combinations for different regions. This has not yet been done. Why?

The reasons behind this are unclear. The WHO is committed to expanding the use of DOT, and many of the most influential experts in the field, from Michael Iseman and John Sbarbaro at Denver, Colorado; Thomas Frieden, previously of New York, now in India; and Arata Kochi, director of the Global Tuberculosis Program, are all firmly committed to DOT. One cannot help wonder whether ideological persuasion does not play a part. DOT programs, when adequately financed and supported, enhance the clinician's authority and increase the public health official's credibility. Whereas fixed-dose combination treatment is almost certainly as effective at controlling the development of drug resistance in comparison with DOT, the absolutist control over disease is not so apparent. "Zero tolerance" of tuberculosis is a notion that flatters DOT programs, with the ultimate sanction (at least in the United States) of detention adding weight, whereas the use of fixed-dose combination treatment fails this test. Treatment compliance is more uncertain, and physician authority is diminished. Detention because of noncompliance with fixed-dose drug treatment regimens is a more difficult concept to argue. Because the risk of relapse may be relatively high with this approach, the risk of relapse with drug-resistant disease is not, and therefore the magnitude of the threat (from MDRTB) is smaller. And it is drug-resistant tuberculosis rather than tuberculosis per se that provokes societal and professional anxiety.

Morally this is a complex issue. The American approach (supported by the WHO) advocates DOT. But ironically, this removes patients' autonomy and replaces it with a paternalistic, authoritarian system.

This, from the nation where autonomy is king. With whatever approach is used, the burdens on the individual need to be weighed against the benefits to the individual. But the burdens of society also must be taken into account. Whereas in New York perhaps, society is prepared to shoulder little additional burden from individuals unprepared, or incapable, of complying with treatment, in other cultural arenas, in other societies, that burden may be willingly shouldered. Elsewhere an "absolutist" approach to control, whereby noncompliance is not tolerated, may itself not be tolerated. Indeed such an approach might be morally unacceptable and as a consequence, in the long-term, be counterproductive as well.

As global policy on tuberculosis is being pushed in the direction of universal DOT, sanctions when DOT is not complied with will be demanded, thus shifting emphasis away from the real goal, that of tuberculosis control and the prevention of drug resistance, to a secondary goal, that of policing treatment compliance. Although this may be only a subtle change, it has major civil liberties consequences that are enhanced by the assumption that DOT is the best approach. And this may not be so.

THE LENS OF TUBERCULOSIS

This book uses the lens of tuberculosis control, and in particular the detention of noninfectious individuals, to examine America's response to its most vulnerable and marginalized citizens, and asks the question: Is detention of noninfectious, noncompliant individuals right from ethical, legal, and public health perspectives? The use of detention is evaluated from a contextual standpoint. After all, detention cannot be justified or condemned in the abstract—the appraisal of such a measure is dependent on situation in which it is occurring.

In chapters 2 and 3 I briefly describe the nature of coercion, the historical and cross-cultural use of this tool in the public health arena, and describe the decline of New York City's model tuberculosis control program. In addition, I describe the social transformation of the city, highlighting the factors that both encouraged the epidemic and hindered the response. In the 1980s and early 1990s, New York City was in the thrall of a tuberculosis epidemic unknown in the developed world since before the introduction, 50 years earlier, of effective antituberculosis drugs. By 1990, with 3 percent of the country's population, the city was accounting for 15 percent of the country's tuberculosis cases. And, across the city, some 40 percent of patients with tuberculosis were failing to complete their treatment, while in some areas the figure was almost 90 percent.[32] In addition, and of perhaps even greater concern than the overall numbers of cases of tuberculosis, large numbers of people had developed strains of disease that were drug resistant and considerably more difficult to treat. These individuals with multidrug-resistant tuberculosis personified for many the change from a curable disease affecting the dispossessed to what was potentially an epidemic of a virtually untreatable casually communicable disease that threatened everyone. Poor compliance was considered to be at the heart of the epidemic.

To address the problem of poor compliance, the state's authority was expanded and a variety of other measures were taken. The city's public health codes were amended to give the commissioner of health the authority to detain noncompliant, noninfectious individuals for long periods. Since 1993, when the amended regulations were adopted, more than 200 noninfectious patients have been detained on Roosevelt Island, some for more than two years. This approach represented a radical shift in the civil liberties/public health balance. In chapter 4 I describe the measures taken and explore the reasons why such an approach was thought necessary. In addition, I examine the ethical underpinning of the law that enables those recalcitrant individuals to be detained. In New York (although not everywhere else in the United States), alternative, less restrictive approaches need not be used before detention is resorted to. This, I suggest, is immoral, lacking in common sense, and probably unconstitutional.

In chapter 5 I describe the effect of the public health program on tuberculosis control in the city and also note how many of the social schisms that were at the heart of the public health emergency persist and may be worsening.

Coercion has been deemed a necessary weapon in the armamentarium of those authorized to protect the public health since before public health fell under the remit of physicians and out of the grip of "sanitarians" and civil engineers. Clearly, from an ethical perspective, coercion is right and necessary on occasion where the public health is threatened. Certainly this is morally justified, at least from a utilitarian standpoint, if the gains (or benefits) to society outweigh the losses. But what if the threat to society is small or, even more problematic, unquantifiable? Since much of the argument for the common good over individual rights is presented in the form of risk assessment, we need to understand what the risks are and what factors influence our perception of those risks. In chapter 6 and 7 I examine the nature of risk, how its perception distorts policy responses, and how cultural and moral mores further influence, and constrain, policy decisions. These chapters provide an analysis of the anxiety created and policy responses provoked by a casual airborne contagion and describe the complex interrelationships among the media, the public, politicians, public health officials, and clinicians. I describe how the response to the epidemic resulted from a distortion of what little objective evidence of risk there was and relied on the perception of public health threat, and I examine the ethical implications of this on public health policymaking. Inextricably intertwined with policymaking are cultural norms, value systems, and attitudes. How these influence responses to those on the margins is an important element to understand when we consider transposing similar approaches to culturally and politically different regions of the world.

In the final two chapters I attempt to draw lessons from the New York City experience, and offer warning and guidance to European public health policymakers and the body politic. With Europe entering an uncertain phase and with a "fortress" mentality developing, those most marginalized, in particular refugees and asylum seekers from areas of the world where communicable diseases are endemic, face an increasingly hostile reception. Added to this increasing public anxiety (fueled by the media) and a newfound political enthusiasm for emphasizing personal responsibility above societal obligations, it is clear that Europe, like the United States, is departing politically from the liberal stance of the 1960s and 1970s. Therein lies the irony in communicable disease control. While autonomy is given still greater prominence over doctors' paternalism, that autonomy is restricted when a public health threat is perceived. Yet society also has responsibilities. It must be fair and just. If it is not, it breeds hopelessness, futility, and hostility—it breeds recalcitrance and noncompliance (in the broader sense of the word). Europe, like the United States, must recognize this. Ultimately our approach to those with communicable diseases reflects on our society, the burden we are prepared to bear in support of patient autonomy, our perceptions of those living on the margins, and our commitment to supporting our most vulnerable members. The contemporary tale of tuberculosis control in New York City, and everywhere else too, is as much a tale of morality and values as it is of medicine.

2

Coercion and the Public Health

The reforms of one generation become the scandals of the next.

—David Rothman, *Conscience and Convenience:*
The Asylum and Its Alternatives in Progressive America, 1971

There has always been tension between the protection of the civil liberties of individuals and the protection of the public health. The state has a role to play in both maintaining and protecting freedom and a role in protecting its citizens from threats to their health. Society's political and moral position on these two areas has been reflected in the legislative response. In the liberal era of the 1960s and 1970s, somewhat draconian approaches to the mentally ill, for example, were questioned and found wanting. Legislation was amended to put patients at the center, to emphasize their rights, and to provide them with greater legal protections. Detention of the mentally ill became dependent on a determination of the threat posed either to themselves or others, and more rigorous legal protections from abuse were provided. Historically a similar approach to isolation of those with communicable diseases also has been taken; detention of individuals with notifiable diseases has been dependent on an assessment of the threat such individuals pose to public health.

Fortunately, the ripples of liberty and health rarely cross. It is infrequent that liberty must be curtailed to enhance health, and vice versa. But when these ripples do cross, turbulence results. Opinions on where the balance lies are influenced as much by political ideology, cultural perspective, and views on morality as by science. Libertarians oppose arguments for increased state interference, and liberal progressives usually oppose the views of moral conservatives. Tuberculosis control highlights these differences par excellence, and in late-twentieth-century New York City, everyone, from policymakers and politicians, to those riding the subway, is concerned about the dangers of this third world disease becoming an uncontrollable epidemic in this greatest of all "first world" cities. The arguments that ensued and the responses of city officials (which culminated in, and were exemplified by, the amendment in 1993 of the city's public health codes) illustrated all these tensions. Tuberculosis, because of the casual nature of its transmission, is as much a social disease, a political disease, as it is medical disease.[1]

Tuberculosis, perhaps more than any other disease, is a lens through which society can be viewed. All of humanity can be examined, from the actions of the dispossessed (who are often those most likely to get the disease), to the responses of the affluent commuters from the suburbs (who are least likely). All are affected by tuberculosis in some way.

Responses reflect how society views those on the margins, from the homeless, drug users, and the HIV-infected, to immigrants and felons. When an epidemic develops, the disease shows how a political and social system works and how a healthcare system responds to a crisis. The threat of potentially untreatable tuberculosis, moreover, increases the power of the lens. When behavioral change is required, how society encourages this reflects as much on society as it does on the irresponsible individual who is failing to comply with treatment. An examination of the New York City tuberculosis epidemic illustrates how a city and a nation respond culturally to a threat.

In many ways the use of coercive public health measures both defines the response to tuberculosis and illustrates a wider societal response to health hazards. In the past many public health physicians sympathized with the suggestion that physicians should welcome the "scientific" approach to disease control "unswervingly without being sidetracked by considerations of social policy."[2] The use of detention as a coercive public health measure in the control of tuberculosis cannot, however, be understood with reference purely to "medicine" or indeed "law," but takes place within the larger field of power and social structure. I reflect in this book, therefore, on questions of American culture and how these influence societal responses. I consider the tensions between personal liberty and social responsibility and place them in the context of tuberculosis control. When are people free to be "recalcitrant" regarding treatment of an airborne infectious disease? How should society respond to those who apparently pose a threat? When does paternalism become excessive? What rules should guide us in our response to those who threaten us with a potentially untreatable disease? Ultimately an understanding of the cultural, social, legal, and ethical perspectives is important to position the use of coercion in the wider arena of public health, to allow lessons to be learned, and to inform future policymaking.

COERCION DEFINED

Coercion can be defined as the act of compelling someone to do something by the use of power, intimidation, or threats. It is a complex concept that covers a wide range of meanings, from the subtle to the overt, from friendly persuasion, to interpersonal pressure, to control of resources, to use of force.[3] For example, some would suggest the doctor-patient relationship is inherently coercive because the power interplay between the two parties is unequal. Clearly, covert, unspoken influences define the relationship and influence the outcome. At the other end of the spectrum are explicit threats of detention unless compliance ensues, whether through changes in behavior as it pertains to the mentally ill or compliance with treatment in the field of tuberculosis control. Just as coercion can be explicit, it may be implied and allied to gentler approaches and other forms of leverage. A threat may be supported, or mollified, by other measures. For example, assistance with finding (and keeping) housing, or a job, may be offered, with the unspoken threat that it may be removed if compliance is not adequate. Unfortunately, little research has been done to examine how subtleties of coercion and leverage influence behavior.

Coercion is frequently used as a pejorative term, suggesting that coercion always demeans individuals who are coerced, and kills their autonomy. Yet to take this view discounts all paternalism and suggests coercion is never just. But this is not so. Many patients who ultimately ended up detained on New York's Roosevelt Island said they were grateful, in the end, to the city. For some, their health and life expectancy had improved immeasurably. For others, the chaos of their lives had been transformed into a calm in which they could reflect upon their life's course. Others (and perhaps the majority) not surprisingly felt the pain of coercion more than the benefit.[4] Few policymakers (or ethicists) would argue that coercion is not justified in order to remove a public health threat given an explicit, defined threat. Indeed, most would say it was unethical not to remove such a threat.

This book uses the term "coercion," in the context of tuberculosis control, to mean "forced action," where the state is involved and sanctions the measures that are implemented. I particularly focus on the use of detention of noninfectious tuberculosis patients, both because this seems to me to be the most extreme use of coercion, falling at one end of the spectrum, and because, as the least restrictive measure available when it is used, it presumably reflects on alternative approaches that have failed to ensure compliance. Coercion in this scenario highlights the extreme measures ultimately required to persuade some individuals to comply with treatment. I also examine the need for coercion in this setting because patients frequently fail to comply, and because many physicians, like myself, who have on occasion found some persistently noncompliant patients exasperating, will have contemplated the need for and perhaps even wished for the "support" and additional authority the threat of detention offers them. Many physicians will be familiar with the emotions aroused by such cases.

THE LIMITS OF COERCION

What impact did coercion have, or, more specifically, what impact did detention of noninfectious patients have, on compliance? The answer to this question is difficult. Certainly compliance in those who were detained improved. After all, release from detention, although not legally dependent on compliance with treatment, was and continues to be so in practice, and the vast majority of cases complete treatment while detained. No patient who resisted treatment has been released from detention. What impact the threat of detention had on those beyond Roosevelt Island's shores is less clear. Most physicians felt it was necessary, and, I am sure, most believe the threat encouraged compliance. Yet disentangling the influence of other factors, such as "enablers" that were introduced (food coupons, travel tokens, etc.), improving access to healthcare, and improving continuity of care from inpatient facility to outpatient facility all undoubtedly also played a part in improving treatment completion rates and compliance. In order to try to determine the impact of detention, I turn here to behavioral science research, which I believe sheds some light on the answer.

More than 60 years ago the behavioral psychologist Floyd Allport described what he called the J-curve hypothesis of conforming behavior.[5] He suggested that when a *rule* comes into effect, the statistical distribution of behavior changes and can be described as a J-curve in reverse. His hypothesis and the data supporting it are useful to review in attempting to understand how treatment compliance might have changed in response to the introduction of more explicit rules or regulations. Allport described several examples of conduct change in response to the introduction of rules. His observations of motorists' behavior in two situations, where rules were different, is illuminating. He looked at how their behavior changed when they were approaching a crossroads and were confronted by a stop sign compared to their behavior when the stop sign was absent. In the situation without the stop signs, 17 percent of drivers stopped, 37 percent went across very slowly, 34 percent slowed down slightly, and 12 percent kept going without slowing down at all. This distribution of behavior can be visualized as a bell-shaped curve. In the scenario where stop signs were in place, his observations showed that 75.5 percent of drivers stopped, 22 percent proceeded through at a very slow speed, only 2 percent went across slowing only a little, and less than 1 percent crossed at their original speed without slowing at all. Represented graphically, these results would resemble the letter J in reverse. He presented other data from other situations, for example, attendance at church and clocking-in times at work, that further supported this hypothesis.

Allport argued that when rules are introduced, behavior changes and the spread of response shifts from a bell-shaped distribution curve to a reverse J-curve. He also suggested that, in order to achieve this behavioral transformation, certain prerequisites are required. First, a recognizable purpose must be set; for example, in the setting of tuberculosis control, compliance with treatment. Second, the rule or regulation that is introduced must be clearly understood, such as the 1993 New York City health code amendments. Third, a fairly large proportion of the population must conform to the proscribed act, that is, most people must be able to comply with treatment, and do so, after the regulations are ratified. The changes in tuberculosis control in the early 1990s in New York and elsewhere in the United States achieved these prerequisites. So, on the basis of this evidence, one might assume that, since the introduction of rules alters behavior, compliance with treatment improved as a consequence, at least in part, of the new regulations. But it may not be as simple as this.

The rigor with which the rules are policed and the cultural context in which they are set may also define the response. These issues, policing of regulations and the cultural influence they exert, are exemplified in the public health arena by immunization practice and results. Between 1989 and 1991 the United States witnessed a measles epidemic that affected particularly preschool city children.[6] Earlier guidelines issued by the Centers for Control and Prevention (CDC) suggesting that all children should have completed a schedule of immunization by age 15 to 18 months old had failed to produce an adequate response. Many children who should have been immunized but had not been developed measles. Compliance with the immunization guidance had been poor. (It has been estimated that immunization coverage across the country for two year olds was less than 80 percent, and considerably less in large cities)[7] In school-age children, immunization rates of more than 95 percent were being achieved with the support of regulations mandating immunization before children could be allowed to enter school.[8] Therefore, it was not the introduction of guidelines but the enforcement of laws that determined conformity. But most measles morbidity and mortality occurs before children's second birthday. So although the rules ensured compliance, the time at which compliance was impacting was ineffective. Thus the time at which rules can influence behavior is important.

The issue of immunization practice also highlights other less obvious influences. In the United Kingdom there is no mandate to *explicitly* coerce parents to have their children immunized. Immunization rates for two-year-olds are, according to the Centre for Disease Surveillance and Control (CDSC), 93 percent and at similar levels in most other European countries.[9] Coercion, or at least recourse to the law, is unnecessary to achieve conformity, which suggests that other factors play an important role. What might these be? We can assume, I think, that parents in Britain and the United States all love their children, want what is best for them, and equally want to protect them from harm. So other factors must be influencing compliance. Access to care is one obvious area. Historically parents in the United States who failed to have their children immunized were likely to be poor and have poor long-term healthcare provision. In the United Kingdom, by contrast, most families have a long-term relationship with a family doctor, the main provider of child healthcare. Another possibility is the media attention and parental anxiety relating to possible adverse reactions from immunizations. Certainly immunization rates fell in the United Kingdom when national attention was focused on the potential of side effects from mumps immunization. But this effect was short-lived, and there is little evidence that low immunization rates in the United States occurred because of active withdrawal of children from immunization programs. It seems that poor immunization coverage arose because of passive neglect. Therefore, the accessibility of healthcare may determine, to some extent, behavior. Cultural differences, discussed in chapter 7, may also play an important role. In his book *Free to Be Foolish,* Howard Leichter illustrates some differences separating the British from their American cousins, including their responses to regulations. He describes, for example, the debate regarding the introduction of mandatory seat-belt use in the two countries: "The point was raised in the course of the debate [in the British Parliament] over mandatory seat-belt use when some opponents argued that the law would be virtually unenforceable and highly unpopular. Proponents countered that the British were a law-abiding people and the measure would be virtually self-enforcing. And it was. The compliance rate has been consistently around 95 percent, compared to about 40 to 50 percent in most American states with compulsory seat-belt laws."[10] Thus, the response to similar rules may produce very different responses depending on the cultural context.

The difficulty in simply translating Allport's model of behavioral change in response to rules in other situations, for example, compliance with antituberculosis treatment, is that the model fails to take account of other influences that may affect behavior. Moreover, it does not explain the reason behind behavioral deviations. An abstract example may be useful to further explore the issue of deviance. If the road on which Allport's crossroads was situated was en route to an emergency trauma unit, we would not be surprised that the proportion of people stopping completely at the junction was small. Even if a stop sign was placed at the crossroads, we would not expect the conformity that would be seen if the crossroads merely served residential streets. Behavior would have been modified in response to the trauma unit. Yet information about the citing of the trauma unit and its impact on traffic behavior would not come across in Allport's simple statistical model. Similarly, while it is clear that compliance with antituberculosis treatment improved when DOT, DOT commissioner's orders, and the threat of detention were introduced, it seems possible that simply improving the access of the service to patients and improving liaison between the hospital and outpatient facilities for follow-up were, in fact, the critical steps taken and that the impact of the regulations was negligible.

Even if one believes that the introduction of the threat of detention was important in influencing compliance and altered the shape of the compliance curve, shifting it from a bell-shaped distribution to a reverse J-curve, one should not have been surprised that some recalcitrant individuals still occupied the tail of the J. Indeed, the tail of the J in many of Allport's experiments was similar to the right-hand tail of the bell. For example, in one of his examples, those who were late for work when there was no "rule" continued to be tardy after rules were imposed. The introduction of rules hardly made an impact on the "hardened recalcitrant," whose behavior continued largely unchanged. Those who fall into the tail of the J do not fall there by chance. When the right-hand tail of the bell-shaped curve is long, the tail of the J-curve can also be expected to be long. That is, the imposition of rules affects the behavior of most, particularly those most prone to comply, but those who were "recalcitrant" before rules were introduced frequently continue to be so. How long the tail of the bell (or, for that matter, the J) stretches, how many individuals are recalcitrant, and why they are is, in essence, a significant part of what I explore in this book. Society, I believe, determines the shape of the bell and the tail of the J. The impact that the threat of detention had on compliance may have influenced treatment compliance of some patients, particularly those who normally would fall within the right-hand slope of the bell curve. But likewise, other changes, in particular access to and provision of care, also may have effected similar change. And for those "hardened" recalcitrant patients, the threat of detention may have achieved little in modifying their behavior. Other societal factors determine the size of that pool of the population. Cultural and societal factors play a substantial part in determining the degree of recalcitrance, deciding how much deviant behavior that society will tolerate, and defining that society's response.

COERCION: A PUBLIC HEALTH TOOL

Three areas deserve to be looked at briefly before we move on to look at contemporary tuberculosis policy in detail. All illustrate a common theme, that of coercion in public health practice, and all offer a historical perspective that helps, I believe, to illuminate contemporary U.S. responses, and therefore future Western responses, to the tuberculosis epidemic. Each area illustrates an arena of public health in which coercion was deemed a necessary resource.

In the next sections I describe the history of vaccination in Britain and the United States to show how a divergence of policies in two Western countries can occur despite some cultural similarities in the perceived public health need to begin with and how ultimately different legal and societal approaches aim to enhance compliance. Furthermore, these historical stories illustrate how apparently coercive measures can be viewed as noncoercive by some, who see policies from a different cultural perspective. Many Americans, even experts in public health, do not think compulsory immunization is a particularly coercive measure. This was somewhat of a surprise to me, having had firsthand experience of what I took to be quite a coercive system. On our arrival in the United States I had not wanted my eldest son, Joe, aged five years, to have an additional immunization against *Haemophilus influenzae* type B (HiB). There was, to my mind, no compelling evidence that a fourth immunization (he had already had three shots in Britain) offered any further protection, and anyway, *H. influenzae* meningitis was, to my knowledge, only a real problem in toddlers. But I was advised that schools cannot legally admit a child who has not been immunized.[11] After some thought I acquiesced; Joe was immunized again and he could go to school, and I could work! I had been surprised by my work colleagues' (at Columbia University, New York) demure acceptance of the public health mandate to coerce immunizations. They, I could tell, were surprised by my reaction, my concern that I was not convinced of the evidence to support the need for additional immunizations and by the fact that I viewed the threat of my child being barred from attending school as coercive. Surely, they said, it was a necessary public health measure to simply ensure good immunization coverage. As can be seen, it is important to gain a cultural appreciation of what is viewed as coercive (and what is not) and an understanding of societal context and the perceived need for such measures.

Next I review the history of detention of mentally ill persons. The mentally ill, even when they pose no threat to others or have committed no crime, have, historically, often been viewed as dangerous and "deranged." In the United States, as elsewhere, commitment of the mentally ill (like commitment for those with tuberculosis) can be seen as a touchstone for how society manages its most vulnerable and "difficult" members. An examination of this area shows us the impact the liberal era and the civil rights movement had on public health. Sociopolitical developments of the 1960s led to the questioning of draconian public health measures that incarcerated many mentally ill patients for years for no good purpose. The new approach put patients at the center of policymaking concerns, emphasized their rights, and asked society to respond accordingly. This approach to detention is at variance in one important respect to detention regulations for tuberculosis patients enacted two decades later. In the 1970s involuntary commitment of the mentally ill became dependent on a determination of the threat they posed to themselves or others—the public health, not their compliance with treatment. More recently, since the shootings of two police officers by a paranoid schizophrenic man at the Capitol in Washington, D.C., some have called for, in addition to better community services, an approach analogous to that used in tuberculosis control: the threat of sanctions if compliance with treatment is not adequate. An about-face may occur. Detention of mentally ill persons was initiated in the mental health arena on the basis of the threat to posed to the public health, and detention of those with tuberculosis followed similar principles. Subsequently detention of tuberculosis patients hinged on the issue of compliance with treatment; control of the mentally ill, it appears, may follow similar notions.

The history of tuberculosis control in the United States, and in particular in New York City, which was at the forefront of earlier reforms, illustrates several parallels with later responses. These included strong leadership and a struggle to gain credibility by public health officials that coincided with the introduction of coercive measures; persisting tensions between clinicians, particularly those in private practice, and public health doctors; and weak or unsupported leadership corresponding to a period of financial and administrative neglect. When the threat of "overspill" of disease from the poor was perceived to be great, coercive measures were assumed to reduce this risk. Little evidence was put forward to substantiate these claims, however. In essence, similar solutions were sought for very similar problems. The brief description of tuberculosis control policy that follows shows that the seeds of the public health failings were sown decades before any noticeable rise in rates occurred, and the response could have been predicted from past approaches.

One common thread runs through all of these public health areas, vaccination and immunization, mental illness, and the historical approach to tuberculosis. Coercion began with those who were least able to protest or resist: children, the mentally ill, and the poor. And alternatives, unless forced by popular mandate, were rarely considered.

VACCINATION POLICY

It was in Britain during the nineteenth century and early twentieth century, while experiencing increased industrialization, that government intervention in the area of public health was first aggressively pursued. The response in the United States mirrored that seen across the Atlantic. Why was this? Despite a lack of history of state paternalism in Britain, there was a long history of aristocratic paternalism. And the changing nature of the relationship between workers and the aristocracy was coincident with the time of increasing urbanization and devastating infectious disease epidemics of cholera, smallpox, scarlet fever, and measles. More endemic, but still a major public health concern, were the thousands of deaths that resulted from tuberculosis and dysentery. The demographic shifts resulting from industrialization resulted in cities growing rapidly. This influx of people into cities, and its associated poverty, caused terrible overcrowding and, in large parts of many cities, appalling living conditions. With poor water supplies, nonexistent sewerage, unsanitary burial procedures and disposal of rubbish, disease, not surprisingly, was rife. Similar social changes were occurring elsewhere in Europe and America.

The unsavory living and working conditions of the poor might have offended the eye (and the nose) of the more genteel classes and have outraged the moral sensibilities of some, but it was for somewhat different, more pragmatic reasons that a government response was demanded. First, disease emanating from the poor threatened the health of the other, more well-to-do classes. Infectious diseases were indiscriminate. Second, the overall health of the population, and men in particular, was a concern because of war. Healthy men were needed to fight in the Crimean (1853-56), Boer (1899-1902), and Great (1914-18) wars. The dawn of microbiological understanding and the advancement of "sanitary science" prompted the state to respond in the ways that it did. Although healthy fighting men were not needed in 1990s New York, the threat of "overspill" was what gave the response its urgency rather than a sudden political concern for the "downtrodden."

Widespread vaccination was part of that historical response. But it was controversial and highlighted early the "subtle art of the administratively possible" that was, and continues to be, at the heart of public health policy promotion where individual freedoms are threatened.[12] Mandatory vaccination was opposed vigorously on both sides of the Atlantic. Vocal antivaccination organizations arose that forced governments to face up to difficult medical, political, and cultural questions.

In Britain, for example, playwright George Bernard Shaw attempted to highlight the risks when he called vaccination "nothing short of attempted murder."[13] Another critic, in attempting to bring attention to the question of the intrusiveness of the state, commented with less florid language that "the political question which it involves is also the largest, because it forces every family in the state to a compliance unlike anything else in the domain of politics."[14] This opposition to the imposition of vaccination initially galvanized the government to strengthen the authority of the Compulsory Vaccination Acts, such that by 1871, the high point in terms of coercion, parents refusing to have their children vaccinated faced imprisonment.

Ironically, it was around the time that John Stuart Mill published *On Liberty* (1859) that the freedom of the individual was curtailed most by the state in the name of public health. And this at a time of economic laissez-faire, when free trade and individualism were at a zenith. While Mill was arguing for the priority of the individual over the authority of the state and society, legislators were attempting to secure "the greatest happiness of the greatest number" and introducing substantially coercive measures. The state's paternalism, along with the crusading fervor of the "public hygiene" movement and the encouragement of many in the medical profession (which was split on the issue) initially disarmed and overcame the opposition.

In Britain those opposing vaccination came from several different quarters, including the medical profession, religious organizations, the Tory press (which opposed Whig paternalism), and the vocal Anti-Vaccination League, founded in 1867. Opposition to vaccination arose principally for four reasons. First, many did not believe the measure was effective at preventing smallpox. Second, many felt that the consequences (including ulceration and, on occasion, fatalities) were sometimes worse than the disease itself. Third, the introduction of a foreign agent into the body, particularly the cowpox vaccine, was sinful and against the laws of God. Last, and of particular interest here, was the opposition that arose from the belief that vaccination threatened personal freedom, that vaccination "unspeakably degrades the freeborn citizen, not only depriving him of liberty of choice in a personal matter, but even denying him the possession of reason."[15] In a similar vein the Tory newspaper, the *Herald*, in opposing intervention, had suggested "a little dirt and freedom, may after all be more desirable than no dirt at all and slavery."[16]

Ultimately, with the opposition to vaccination persisting, and with divisions within both government and the organized medical profession running deep, the 1871 act was watered down such that following the 1907 act, parents could exempt their children by providing a written declaration of opposition to a justice of the peace.[17] In effect, this is what persists today. Currently, in England and Wales, regulation 10 of the 1988 Public Health (Infectious Diseases) Act permits the health officer, "if he considers it in the public interest, [to] arrange for the vaccination or immunisation, without charge, of any person in his district or port health district who has come or may have come or may come in contact with the infection *and is willing* to be vaccinated or immunised."[18] Coverage these days for immunizations and vaccinations is good, with over 90 percent of children being vaccinated by the time authorities recommend.[19]

The same questions and arguments surrounding the imposition of vaccination that surfaced in Britain also arose in America at around the same time, but because of the federal nature of the United States there were, and are, no national vaccination regulations, although there are federal guidelines. Instead, states responded independently, and often differently, each enacting its own legislation. For example, Utah had a complete prohibition of vaccination in the nineteenth century while, by 1850, five states had made vaccination either compulsory or optional.[20] Not surprisingly, opposition varied considerably between states, but as in Britain, lobbying through pamphlets and organizations was noisy.

In 1905 the U.S. Supreme Court ruled on the issue. A Mr. Jacobson had refused to have his child vaccinated in response to a smallpox outbreak in Massachusetts, claiming that both he and his child had previously had adverse reactions. The state had contested his decision, and the case had reached the Supreme Court. In the ruling the Court upheld the constitutionality of compulsory vaccination and dismissed concerns regarding efficacy and side effects. But the Court "refrained from any attempt to define the limits of [police] power"[21] and left that decision up to the individual states. The Court did, however, give vague guidance: "[T]he police power of a state must be held to embrace, at least, such reasonable regulations established directly by legislative enactment as will protect the public health and the public safety."[22] Public health safety, therefore, overrode concerns regarding efficacy and potential harm arising from vaccination and bowed to medical expertise to define the limits of threat the public might be willing to accept.

Jacobson v. Massachusetts also helped to clarify whether vaccination was an invasion of liberty or "unreasonable, arbitrary, and oppressive and, therefore, hostile to the inherent right of every freeman to care for his own body and health in such way as to him seems best."[23] The Court decided vaccination was not an invasion of liberty, or if it was, then the public health benefits overrode that intrusion. *Jacobson* was a landmark case. It determined, however vaguely, that the common good, the public health, outweighed individual freedom, and it gave government the authority to restrict freedom.[24] What it did not do, however, was define the boundaries where government intervention is reasonable (and constitutional) and where it is not.

The history of vaccination in Britain and the United States highlights differences in societal approach from similar initial nine-teenth-century responses. In the United States explicit coercion has persisted as a public health tool whereas in Britain, a purportedly more deferential nation with a stronger paternalistic tradition, the coercive elements were repealed. Similar approaches have, broadly, been adopted elsewhere in western Europe.[25] This European-American divergence arose at the turn of the century and has persisted, I believe, for a number of reasons. In Britain the state responded to opposition by revoking nationally applicable legislation. In the U.S. federal system, a piecemeal implementation of vaccination policy had occurred, and a national response was unnecessary. The opposition varied in intensity from state to state. The power of the antivaccination lobby (with members of Parliament, the upper classes, and much of the medical profession opposed) was perhaps stronger and more vociferous in the United Kingdom. And the subsequent development of the welfare state and, in particular, the National Health Service enabled almost all of the population to have easy access to a family doctor who provided long-term ongoing care for families. The strength of the doctor-patient relationship, even in cities and among the poor, meant overt (although not necessarily covert) coercion was unnecessary. As the epidemics and mortality rate of childhood diseases were waning, as public faith in immunization as a preventive tool rose, and as public attention was diverted to other more pressing concerns, the pressure to look again at the legislation fell. Finally, the differences in approach underlie some important cultural differences that are relevant in the wider consideration of coercion as a public health tool. First, the role of the law to support public health actions and the sanctions that can be imposed if compliance is poor are clear in the United States. In Britain a voluntary code is used. Second, the increased use of formal regulations encourages an absolutist approach, whereby nonconformity or noncompliance is more difficult "to get away with" where sanctions can be imposed, but such an approach may be less successful when they cannot. In their book *The Perversion of Autonomy,* Willard Gaylin and Bruce Jennings, two ethicists from The Hastings Center in New York, decry the absurdities that can follow when autonomy is made sacrosanct.[26] They argue that other moral principles should receive equal, if not greater, attention. I agree. The ethical question, it seems, is where that balance lies. In their book the authors call for intimidation or coercion in vaccination policy so that "Harlem children be protected." They remark that "There is something immoral about spending millions, even hundreds of millions, of dollars on programs to 'educate' people to change their behavior, when we know that what is necessary is either intimidation or coercion." The certainty of these views is striking. Have the authors failed to look beyond U.S. shores at the great public health successes achieved without intimidatory methods? While they claim that education may be a waste of time and money, overt coercion is not the only alternative. Structural societal change should also be considered. The immorality of failing to offer decent universal healthcare services to society's poorest and youngest seems to me a greater injustice, and apparently one not contemplated before coercive measures are reached for.

INVOLUNTARY COMMITMENT OF THE MENTALLY ILL

In late-nineteenth-century America, the commitment of the mentally ill was straightforward. Most states afforded few, if any, legal protections to those threatened with commitment. Indeed, anyone could request an individual be committed for an indefinite time. Housewives could be committed by their husbands for neglecting their housework.[27] It was against this background that reformers sought to introduce protections for patients and to prevent inappropriate commitments. But during the first half of the twentieth century, few protections for the mentally ill existed. During this period psychiatric institutions were expanding dramatically in response to reformers' beliefs that institutions could solve social ills, including crime, mental illness, and poverty. This was abetted by the promotion of the medical model, which "rests on the assumption that some mentally ill persons are unable to control their dangerous behavior or are too cognitively impaired to recognize their need for treatment."[28] In most states commitment was for an indefinite period. Most patients, once committed, stayed institutionalized for years. For example, by 1937 the average length of hospital confinement was more than nine years.[29] By 1955 there were more than 800,000 inpatients in state and county mental hospitals across the country.[30]

The shift away from institutionalization for the mentally ill started in the mid-1950s, when a presidential commission suggested that the aim of modern care should be to maintain individuals in the community. This change in direction occurred largely because of financial concerns over the cost of such massive institutionalization but also because of concerns that patients were not benefiting from their treatment (and might even be being harmed), and civil rights concerns.[31] The policy move to deinstitutionalization was formalized with the passage of The Mental Retardation Facilities and Community Mental Health Center Construction Act in 1963.

In the late 1960s and early 1970s activist lawyers acting on behalf of mentally ill persons argued in federal courts that involuntary commitment should be understood not as a state activity that benefits the mentally ill but as an action that removes a fundamental right of liberty that is deserving of constitutional protection. They argued that "the only state interest sufficiently compelling to permit preventive detention was the prevention of harm."[32] In 1972, in a landmark case, a federal district court struck down a Wisconsin statute as unconstitutional because it permitted nondangerous mentally ill individuals to be forcibly detained.[33] Other courts followed suit (New York, for example, in 1975) and limited forcible commitment of the mentally ill to those who posed a threat of harm. This threat of harm now has to be shown "by clear and convincing evidence," and to justify commitment the danger posed must be "imminent" or "in the near future."[34] The state may not, the Supreme Court later noted, just "fence in the harmless mentally ill solely to save its citizens from exposure to those whose ways are different. . . . The State cannot constitutionally confine . . . a nondangerous individual who is capable of surviving safely in freedom by himself or with the help of willing and responsible family friends and family."[35]

Since the 1970s the detention of the mentally ill, therefore, has hinged on a determination of the danger individuals are to themselves or to the public. And the authorities, the courts decided, cannot simply detain an individual who refuses treatment. It must also be determined that he "lacks sufficient insight to make a responsible decision."[36]

Since these changes described occurred, with the end of the liberal era and the advent of the neoconservative era of Presidents Ronald Reagan and George Bush (and Bill Clinton), the broad policy approach has changed again. It has shifted toward enveloping the mentally ill in the criminal justice system. Mental illness has been "criminalized," because of the failure to adequately support fledgling community care programs and the fear generated within communities from the rise in homelessness, "psychiatric ghettos," and the disappearance of safe havens for the seriously disturbed.[37] As lawyer Nancy Rhoden noted in regard to judicial support for the mentally ill: "Since judicial decrees can grant rights against government infringement of liberty far more easily than they can establish positive entitlements to care and services, the result was that mental patients obtained their liberty, but at the expense of the community care they so desperately needed."[38] Many mentally ill persons have found themselves in neither mental institutions nor cared for in the community but in prisons and jails for often minor misdemeanors and drug-related crimes. Not surprisingly, the criminal justice system, like its predecessor, has failed to control the behavior of the mentally ill individuals who did not meet the liberal era's statutory commitment requirements. Mass institutionalization in mental health facilities (as well as in prisons) is occurring again, and expansion of mental institutions is progressing rapidly. Again, as in the progressive era, this is being done under the cover of altruism, a paternalistic approach that purportedly protects patients from themselves, but also rids communities of the insane, the homeless, those whom others feel uncomfortable being around, although they pose no threat to anyone beyond themselves. Since 1979 several states have changed their laws to permit involuntary commitment of mentally ill individuals in need of treatment who are not necessarily dangerous even to themselves.[39] The pendulum is swinging back away from autonomy, but the arc has been somewhat deflected. While the utilitarian harm principle determined early-twentieth-century policies toward the mentally ill, those policies also were colored substantially by potent beneficent, paternalistic principles. These, it could be argued, were sacrificed to the illusion of autonomy in the liberal era. Now autonomy, it might be said, is being sacrificed on a distorted Benthamite altar where the perceived harm that the mentally ill pose to others is insufficiently tempered by paternalistic, beneficent principles.

This change has been illustrated in the debate regarding Russell E. Weston, the suspect in the fatal shootings of two police officers in the Capitol building. A paranoid schizophrenic, he had fallen through the sizable gaps in the community network that was meant to provide care for him. Many experts are suggesting that with adequate community support individuals like Mr. Weston could have been helped and the course of events been altered. Others are complaining, however, that the problem is not that inadequate support is given but that the laws allowing the mentally ill to be detained involuntarily are too "tough," that the legal emphasis on a determination of the threat such a person poses is too uncertain to enable commitment. Some people (at present in a minority) are calling, therefore, for measures analogous to those introduced in response to the tuberculosis epidemic; that the threat of harm need only be of secondary importance, that compliance with antipsychotic medication should be the first principle of care, and that the threat of involuntary detention can be used to enhance compliance with antipsychotic medication.[40] Indeed in New York "Kendra's Law," named for Kendra Webdale who died after being pushed in front of a subway train by a diagnosed schizophrenic who was not taking his medication, enables the courts to detain non-compliant mentally ill persons if orders to comply with treatment are violated. Although the threat posed by Mr. Weston is at the heart of the debate about how he, and others like him, should be managed, it would, these experts argue, be easier if assessments of the threat he poses are left to one side. Measures of compliance should be used, they argue, to dictate public health responses.

As can be seen from this brief description, approaches to detention of the mentally ill have shifted from 30 years ago when the arbitrary opinion of experts (and the not so expert) dictated the use of coercive measures, to an overemphasis on autonomy, and to an enthusiasm for the immeasurable assessment of the public health threat posed by individuals. Recently, because of popular fear, involuntary commitment (tied to coercive community practices) has again become a useful social engineering tool.[41] There are several similarities (and some differences) with the contemporary tuberculosis control response. With tuberculosis, detention of noninfectious patients now hangs on the concept of compliance. Notions of public health threat, although at the heart of the response, are in large part only alluded to.

Why has detention of noncompliant tuberculosis patients in the 1990s not followed the model of commitment for the mentally ill in the 1970s? In essence this *was* the model adopted up until the New York City epidemic prompted regulatory changes in the early 1990s. In a 1980 West Virginia case, for example, it was noted that the same rationale governing the involuntary commitment of a mentally ill person lay behind the state's Tuberculosis Control Act, that is, to prevent the person becoming a danger to others.[42] The 1959 New York statute had allowed detention "upon determining that the health of others is endangered." Yet, unlike the 1970s, when institutions for the mentally ill were closing and the civil rights movement was in full swing, by the 1990s, although there were concerns over costs and an awareness of civil liberties principles, public health officials and city authorities were much more aware of the uncertainties of risk assessment, particularly with regard to public health. By emphasizing compliance they could quantify behavior and leave the assumption of threat hanging in the air. In addition, in the 1990s the calls for a rapid response were more urgent and louder, the flow of patients was in the opposite direction, coercive measures were being introduced rather than rescinded, and patients were being detained rather than released. Moreover, financial savings were not such a political issue. The threat of the tuberculosis epidemic weighed more heavily on the shoulders of politicians than the cost of the response, and the potential costs in the future because of errors made dwarfed what needed to be spent. Finally, there was an ideological shift in perceptions of societal and personal responsibilities. The inspiration from the Great Society was long past, and in 1993 the wake from Reagan's moral crusade was still strong.

TUBERCULOSIS PUBLIC HEALTH POLICY IN NEW YORK, 1882 TO 1970

By understanding the historical response to the "captain of all these men of death," we can recognize similarities that help to explain later events and indeed the perimeters of future choices. The decisions made in response to the later epidemic were governed, in some measure, by earlier attempts at control. Indeed, the controversies regarding the isolation of patients in the nineteenth and early twentieth century show, just like now, that disputes over matters of science and public health policy were rooted in deep ideological divisions, with libertarians seeking to break the bonds of an overintrusive, paternalistic state while others viewed the stretching of the state's authority more sympathetically.

It is important to remember that public health originated in the nineteenth century from concerns that were initially more sanitary than medical. Only toward the end of the century, as hospitals and public health activities expanded with increasing understanding of disease and "germ theory" and became directly related to medical care, did the system we recognize today begin to take shape. During the Reformation prevalent opinion warned that sin and immorality were predisposing causes of illness; prayer was perceived to be the appropriate, although often insufficient, response. Moral error was considered responsible for disease. These moral undertones, it can be argued, continue to influence our response to disease today. For example, when we compare sex workers or intravenous drug users infected with human immunodeficiency virus with "innocent" children or hemophiliacs, our responses are redolent with moral hand-wringing.

By the mid-nineteenth century, with the increasing recognition of the microbiological etiology of disease, public health organizations using methods arising from a medical approach gained authority, but there was some resistance.[43] Public health authorities shifted attention from the environment to the individual, and they increasingly focused on the techniques of medicine and personal hygiene.[44] This was partly a response to the contagious nature of many diseases. One way to prevent the spread of disease is to diagnose and cure those who are ill. This approach to public health brought public health officials into conflict with physicians, particularly private ones, who were concerned about the extension of public health's boundaries into areas that had been their responsibility and about the erosion of their autonomy and earnings. Physicians opposed public treatment of the sick, communicable disease reporting requirements, and public preventive and curative medical centers. The tensions among public health, the medical profession, and the patient have long been recognized. In the mid-nineteenth century, for example, it was noted by the Metropolitan Board of Health of the State of New York that "The Health Department of a great commercial district which encounters no obstacles and meets with no opposition, may safely be declared unworthy of public confidence; for no sanitary measures, however simple, can be enforced without compelling individuals to yield something of pecuniary interest or of personal convenience to the general welfare."[45] These tensions have persisted and are present to this day.

Physicians' responses to state intervention in the nineteenth century illuminate contemporary views on intervention by the federal government, particularly the response to the Clinton administration's proposed health reform. The medical profession resisted reform in the early 1990s when their autonomy was threatened by political efforts to expand healthcare coverage, but they supported federal intervention in 1999 to ensure quality since their autonomy has been reduced by health maintenance organizations (HMOs). When the extension of states' regulatory powers helped protect their income, for example, by licensing

medical practice in the late nineteenth century, physicians were enthusiastic supporters of intervention. When, however, interventions threatened either their autonomy or income, for example, in encouraging
public dispensaries (for free medicines), then their opposition was
strenuous. As public health extended its remit, resistance from physicians became more pronounced.[46] To some degree New York was
exceptional in that its Public Health Department was very active—in
many areas public health received very little attention.

The historical conflict between public health's responsibilities and
private doctors' concerns was illustrated by the response to the public
health department's initiatives to control tuberculosis. At the time
German bacteriologist Robert Koch first described the tubercle bacillus
in 1882, tuberculosis was the leading cause of death in New York City.
By 1889 the Health Department had accepted that tuberculosis was
both communicable and preventable. In 1893 tuberculosis was added to
the list of communicable diseases, and the Health Department decided
to require the identification within ten days of those persons with
tuberculosis to ensure appropriate care, which at the time included the
disinfection of living quarters and disposal of sputum. Once registered,
cases came under "direct surveillance" from the department's inspectors,
unless physicians agreed "to provide the instruction necessary to prevent
the spread of contagion." Thus physicians were requested to inform the
department of any of their patients with tuberculosis. Free laboratory
services for testing for tuberculosis were offered to encourage reporting
and assist in the identification of cases. Depending on this voluntary
reporting, however, failed, and Hermann Biggs, director of the new
laboratory services and an influential leader in the new public health
arena, promoted the passage of an ordinance on January 19, 1897,
declaring pulmonary (in contrast to extrapulmonary) tuberculosis "an
infectious and communicable disease, dangerous to the public health."[47]
Notification by private doctors was thereafter made mandatory (as it had
been for public institutions and dispensaries).[48] Not surprisingly, private
doctors opposed mandatory reporting, suggesting it was an invasion of
the relationship they held with their patients and of patients' rights to
confidentiality. Furthermore, they felt the ordinance was "offensively
dictatorial and defiantly compulsory."[49] The president of the New York
County Medical Society stated this view in 1897, when he told its
membership that the Health Department was "usurping the duties,

rights and privileges of the medical profession" and called the measure "unnecessary, inexpedient, and unwise."[50] The New York medical profession finally formally recognized the Health Department's policy in 1900.[51] It is unclear how effective these mandatory measures were in increasing reporting, but notification levels did increase.[52] What is clear is that the authority of the public health officials had been extended.

With the encouragement of Hermann Biggs, other cities followed New York's lead.[53] One physician, in support of Biggs's approach, illustrated an acute awareness of class differences and needs when he remarked at the 1900 Philadelphia County Medical Society meeting:

> There is no earthly reason why that individual [with tuberculosis] should not be reported to the authorities as a tubercular subject. His physician should report him, but the individual should not know it; and if this individual occupies a social position that will guarantee intelligent observation of the directions given him by his physicians, there is no earthly reason why the authorities should fear in the least, but unfortunately these physicians cover a very small community. In a very large proportion of the community in which tuberculosis exists and in which it forms a menace to our people who cannot or will not, or perhaps both, follow the directions of the physicians, my belief is, in these cases, the Board of Health should be authorized to look after them, to disinfect the premises.[54]

The doctor concluded by suggesting that those patients with tuberculosis whose social position failed to guarantee "intelligent observation" of their doctor's directives should be made wards of the state and held in sanatoriums.

On reflection, it is remarkable how the wording used nearly a century later in the adoption of regulatory amendments allowing for the detention of those who "can not be relied upon to participate in and/or to complete an appropriate prescribed course of medication for tuberculosis" echoes his words.[55] Furthermore, the implicit observation that those of "elevated" social position need not be policed has a resonance today where care is provided through a private physician rather than through the public chest clinics and the city's Bureau of Tuberculosis Control struggles to monitor and ensure compliance with treatment in these latter cases.

The advent of bacteriology and the resulting improved understanding regarding the infectiousness of some diseases encouraged the move
away from somewhat indiscriminate public health measures advocated
earlier in the nineteenth century. As a result, costs were reduced and
public health officials were distanced from moral judgments (although
they still made moral judgments). In addition, pressures for social
reform were diluted. This new focused, bacteriological approach, therefore, brought with it reduced requirements of public health. For
example, Charles Chapin, like Biggs an influential figure in the field at
the turn of the twentieth century, criticized earlier public health
measures, arguing that they made no "distinction between dangerous
dirt and dirt not dangerous, and warfare was waged against everything
decaying and everything which smelled bad."[56] He, and others, brought
a new scientific rigor to public health through their understanding of
microbiology: "It is only along the line of patient investigation of each
disease and practical deductions from ascertained facts that public health
work can succeed. . . . [W]e must learn the nature and mode of
transmission of each infection, and must discover its most vulnerable
point of attack."[57] However, in focusing narrowly on the microbiological aspects of disease, Chapin decried broad social intervention: "I fail to
see how poor housing in itself produces much disease."

Chapin and his colleagues, therefore, helped put housing and other
broad areas of social reform beyond the remit of public health, despite
both epidemiologic and laboratory evidence suggesting that social
conditions might play an important role in the epidemiology of a disease
like tuberculosis.[58] In 1890 death rates from tuberculosis in a "beautiful
residential" section on the Upper West Side of Manhattan were 49 per
100,000, compared to 776 per 100,000 in the crowded tenements of
lower Manhattan. S. Adolphus Knopf, a renowned social reformer,
described those most likely to develop tuberculosis: Those who were
alcoholics and victims of poverty were most prone, and he suggested
that, through "ignorance or carelessness," they spread the disease
"without any regard to the danger" to others.[59] Knopf and others
showed by their research and in their essays that tuberculosis was
associated with overcrowding, poor nutrition, and alcoholism. He and
other progressive reformers of the time advocated a social agenda that
included remodeling tenement housing, abolishing sweatshops, reducing hours of labor, sterilizing milk, and broadly improving the standard

of living. Tuberculosis, it was well recognized, was more prevalent in poor, overcrowded neighborhoods. Experimental evidence was supporting these social observations.

In a remarkable series of experiments before the turn of the twentieth century, Edward Livingston Trudeau, a doctor who had suffered from tuberculosis, had shown that rabbits deprived of light, fresh air, exercise, and adequate nutrition succumbed more readily to tuberculosis than those treated well.[60] Trudeau divided 15 rabbits into three groups. Group 1 was inoculated with *M. tuberculosis* and then kept in a small box "in a dark cellar . . . deprived of light, fresh air, and exercise," and maintained on small rations. Four of the five rabbits died within three months, and the fourth was found to have a "solidified and shrivelled" lung at autopsy. Group 2 was kept under the same conditions as Group 1 but not inoculated with *M. tuberculosis*. Four months later none had developed disease, but all "were emaciated." The last group, Group 3, was inoculated and released onto a small island where food was widely available. One of these five rabbits died a month after inoculation. The remaining four thrived and at autopsy, as part of the experiment, were free of disease.

Despite the epidemiological and experimental evidence showing the complex factors influencing the development of disease, the reductionist medical model was dominant. Perhaps not by coincidence the narrower medical approach was also more politically acceptable. Just as the tensions among patients, their physicians, and public health officials have persisted, so too have tensions between those advocating broad social reform and those positing a narrower, more politically acceptable approach.

Although the use of coercive measures by health departments had been recognized for some time, at the end of the nineteenth century the emphasis on control of tuberculosis moved toward control of individual behavior, and health departments advocated policies to instruct and supervise those with tuberculosis.[61] Teams of inspectors went out to visit the homes of individuals with tuberculosis, and "verbal instruction . . . about the danger of infection and the care of sputum," sleeping alone, and dietary advice was given.[62] If the family was uncooperative formal procedures were initiated to remove the children and institutionalize the sick. The magnitude of risk was *assumed,* much as it had been a hundred years later. Biggs advanced these coercive measures by stressing that: "the cry has been raised again and again that for humanity's sake pulmonary consumption must not be pronounced a communicable disease, and the friends of patients often declare that they prefer to expose themselves to the chance of infection rather than have their dear ones banished, or treated as if they were plague-stricken; but this is all the sheerest nonsense."[63] Biggs recognized the civil liberties issues in relation to the use of coercive measures but clearly felt the benefits outweighed the costs. He remarked, for example, that "The government of the United States is democratic but the sanitary measures adopted are sometimes autocratic, and the functions performed by sanitary authorities paternal in character. We are prepared, when necessary, to introduce and enforce, and the people are ready to accept, measures which might seem radical and arbitrary, if they were not plainly designed for the public good, and *evidently beneficent* in their effects"[64] (emphasis added). Others, including Chapin, had similar views: "Our business, daily and hourly, leads us to the depletion of men's pockets and the restriction of their liberty. We cannot expect the thanks of those who feel themselves aggrieved."[65] As I shall show, the evidence of benefit from isolation was not clear then nor years, later when similar calls for coercive measures were raised.

Restrictions and other coercive measures were not applied uniformly but rather were focused on the "lower classes." As Henry Sewall, a Denver physician, remarked in 1904: "TB is a respectable disease if you have money, but without it, it is a mean low-down business."[66]

By and large, the medical fraternity was in agreement. In 1896 Dr. Charles Ingraham urged the American Medical Association to promote a network of state hospitals for consumptives where they could be "*sentenced* by health officials for a greater or less term, according to the seriousness and persistence of their *offence*"[67] (emphasis added). Later, in 1907, in an address to the National Association for the Study and Prevention of Tuberculosis, Dr. William Welch commented: "In dealing with patients who are a serious menace to the community, who cannot or will not be taught to take proper safeguards against infection of their fellow-men, I think that the health authorities should be empowered to place them in proper institutions."[68]

Although the language and tone of officials advocating detention may jar today, many of the sentiments expressed were similar to those expressed in the 1980s and early 1990s in New York. In order to pursue public health policy, health officials threatened and used their power to confine those who were "liable to jeopardize the health of others." Most city councils and state legislatures around the turn of the twentieth century considered the commitment of those with tuberculosis "a valid exercise of the police power of the state."[69] Few people protested this use of authority. After all, it was used largely against vagrants, uneducated immigrants, and those without a political voice.

Several health departments, in order to facilitate confinement, dedicated hospital wards or hospitals to the cause of isolation for consumptives. In 1903, for example, Riverside Hospital in New York was designated as the facility for the involuntary confinement of those whose "dissipated and vicious habits" endangered the public health.[70] Historian Sheila Rothman suggests in her book *Living in the Shadow of Death* that Riverside became as much a dumping ground for recalcitrant individuals as a hospital.[71] The facilities at Riverside were, as a consequence, inadequate. In 1914 the superintendent of the hospital noted: "There are neither *police officers* to govern nor *cells* or quiet rooms in which to confine these recalcitrant ones. The only weapons in the hands of the hospital authorities are those of argument or persuasion"[72](emphasis added). Clearly there was uncertainty over whether such institutions were hospitals or prisons. In the end these facilities served as a "place of last resort to the narrow group of cases, in the extreme stages of physical and economic helplessness."[73] Many patients went to them for shelter in the winter. As Rothman noted, what separated these institutions from prisons may have been the proximity of death.[74] They offered a choice: Either stay and be cured, albeit with the sacrifice of dignity, or leave and die. Unfortunately, many stayed and still died undignified deaths from tuberculosis, with the consequent dilution of the medical arguments persuading patients to stay. Bitterness increased and many patients left these facilities against medical advice. By the end of 1918 the New York City Bureau of Preventable Diseases had on record the names of 9,479 individuals with reported tuberculosis who had disappeared from observation and could not be traced. Despite the facts that the numbers of patients far outstripped the facilities provided and many absconded, even as late as 1919 there were still 654 patients classified as "sanitary supervision cases."

With death rates from tuberculosis declining after the turn of the twentieth century, public health measures began to receive less attention.

By 1928 the tuberculosis clinics of New York City's Department of Health were described as inadequate, and it was recommended that private and public hospitals care for tuberculosis patients in their outpatient clinics rather than the department's clinics. At that time it was estimated that one bed should be available for each annual tuberculosis death. New York City, in 1927, suffered 5,157 deaths but had only 3,800 beds.[75] It is illuminating to look ahead 10 years to a *New York Times* article when contemplating the inadequacy of the city's response: "It is a matter of great regret that the Board of Estimate cannot actually behold 30,000 gaunt, emaciated figures, with death gleaming in the eyes of many. These are the tuberculous who are always with the city."[76]

As with the financial crisis of 1975, with the collapse of Wall Street in 1929 and the onset of the Great Depression, tax revenues dried up and the deficit grew, slowing progress toward control of tuberculosis considerably. By 1938 the new health commissioner, J. Haven Emerson, stated in a radio address that the lack of hospital facilities for white tuberculosis patients would be remedied when city finances permitted the completion of the new hospitals proposed by an earlier commissioner, S. Goldwater, but he questioned whether the program would take care of blacks and Puerto Ricans. He concluded: "We have not yet been entirely just and adequate in our public services to the people of the coloured races in our city."[77] He recognized that some sections of New York City were more severely affected than others. One section of the Lower West Side had consistently shown a death rate of 350 or more per 100,000 for 50 years compared to rates of less than a third of that for the city as a whole.[78]

After World War II, with the introduction of antibiotics in the late 1940s, public health circles took on renewed vigor and once again the incarceration of patients with infectious tuberculosis for the public protection gained momentum in the United States. By 1950 public health spending on tuberculosis ranked second, outstripped only by that spent on venereal diseases.[79] It soon became clear that, in order to prevent frequent relapses, particularly those that subsequently did not respond to treatment the second time around, combination treatment was necessary for prolonged periods without interruption. It was recognized shortly after effective drugs became available, in the 1950s, that erratic use of these agents, either because of inadequate healthcare provision or because of poor compliance, appeared to promote resistance.[80]

Death rates from tuberculosis fell further after the introduction of antituberculosis agents. With the optimism brought about by the possibility of a cure, and the concern that this might be jeopardized by those who remained infectious in New York and elsewhere, once again the use of quarantine to control tuberculosis became a focus. For example, Washington State redrafted its public health legislation to enable health officials to quarantine individuals with active tuberculosis who were "uncooperative" and "refused to observe the [necessary] precautions to prevent the spread of disease.'[81] These new regulations gave health officials a great deal of latitude in judging what behavior threatened the public's health.[82]

By 1954 it was clearer than ever that tuberculosis was concentrated in certain city areas and among certain segments of the population. The New York City commissioner at the time strengthened the tuberculosis prevention program by increasing its funding, funding that came from the Bureau of Social Hygiene (which had benefited from the use of penicillin in treating venereal diseases). Recently available treatment allowed outpatient care for many patients who would have previously been hospitalized. In the 1955-56 period the Health Department took 1,172,000 X-rays and uncovered over 3,000 cases of tuberculosis, 90 percent of which had not previously been reported.

Social deprivation continued to persist in some areas throughout this period and accounted for marked differences in tuberculosis rates. For example, 1959 statistics show that death rates in Harlem were over 50 percent higher than for New York City as a whole. Health commissioner L. Baumgartner recommended that the disease be treated "promptly and vigorously," with early institutional care "provided by compulsory methods, if necessary," until patients were noninfectious.[83] Through the 1960s the association between tuberculosis and social deprivation continued. At this time also, recognition dawned in the city of yet another problem that would assume even greater importance in the years to come. In 1962 the tuberculosis bureau noted: "The end of the first decade of oral chemotherapy finds us with one major unsolved problem. Tuberculosis has become even more strikingly than before a disease of the poor, of the slum, the aged, and the minorities." In addition, the report noted that these patients attended clinics irregularly. Moreover, the Department of Health estimated that medical follow-up of many outpatients with active disease was inadequate and that the situation since 1960 had become worse.[84] The bureau commented in a report that the economic and social climate "in which tuberculosis breeds is not favorable to its cure." This report concluded: "During the next decade a massive assault must be directed against the real root of the disease, which is poverty, if substantial progress towards its eradication is to be made."[85]

By 1964, George James, then commissioner of health, estimated that 13,000 deaths during the preceding year were largely attributable to the appalling conditions in which one-fifth of the city's population lived. Like early progressive reformers at the turn of the twentieth century, he suggested that the "outmoded practice of treating the single disease and ignoring the whole man" was insufficient and inappropriate.[86] Others concurred. The Board of Health's Annual Report stated bluntly that New York City had some of the worst medical care in the state and that organized medicine was doing little to help. Although tuberculosis rates continued to decline by about 2 percent a year in the 1960s, the Department of Health, when appealing for federal funds, noted that the rate of disease was climbing in deprived areas, particularly among blacks and Hispanics.[87]

The erratic treatment of patients, which was recognized to be associated with increased relapse rates, was noted in the 1960s to be causing drug resistance in significant numbers of patients. By the 1970s multidrug resistance was a substantial problem. The combined rate of primary and acquired resistance to isoniazid, one of the cornerstone drugs in the treatment of tuberculosis, was 8 percent.[88] Poor compliance was at the heart of the increase in drug resistance. Therefore, the city increased treatment supervision by employing healthcare workers to track down and encourage patients whose treatment was erratic to comply. Noncompliant patients were also detained, although usually for only short periods. From about 3,000 to 4,000 new cases appeared in the city each year. Of these, approximately 80 patients were incarcerated annually in the years leading up to 1970.[89]

The history of tuberculosis up to 1970 in the United States and New York City illuminates many of the sources of the contemporary epidemic, and many of the later responses are mirrored in earlier attempts at control. As emphasis on the "germ theory" of disease was developed, so the individualistic nature of control efforts was advanced, and attempts at societal shaping to promote public health withered. The tensions between public health officials and physicians and patients that was obvious in the past persists to this day and continues to influence policy decisions. When coercive measures were advocated, the perceived magnitude of the tuberculosis threat was amplified beyond what available objective evidence suggested in order to secure support. Finally, political and financial support occurred at times when leadership was enthusiastic and public anxiety had been stimulated. Only when those outside poor neighborhoods felt threatened were substantial control efforts advanced. The seeds of the contemporary epidemic were decades old and could be found in the poverty-stricken areas of the city.

3

The Seeds of an Epidemic

Obviously, the equilibrium between man and the tubercle bacillus is very precarious. If war can so rapidly upset it, other unforeseen events might also cause recurrences of the tuberculosis epidemic in the Western world. . . . In the final analysis, the fight against tuberculosis can be carried along two independent approaches, by preventing the spread of the bacilli through procedures of public health, and by increasing the resistance of man through a proper way of life.

—René and Jean Dubos,
The White Plague: Tuberculosis, Man, and Society, 1952

This chapter highlights the epidemic nature of tuberculosis in New York City from the 1970s to the early 1990s and describes the public health failures and other factors that had an impact on, either directly or indirectly, the tuberculosis problem. Many policies in areas broader than what is commonly construed today as "public health" exacerbated the tuberculosis epidemic, but they also heightened a sense of alienation in individuals who were, during the 1980s, frequently called "the underclass." And it was from this population that many of the "delinquent" patients who were thought to be at "the core of New York City's TB problem" arose, the persistently noncompliant "recalcitrant" patients.[1] These individuals could be found at the end of the compliant-recalcitrant behavioral spectrum. They failed to comply with treatment even after inducements had been introduced, and it was they who aroused fear and were the focus of coercive measures.

INCREASING TUBERCULOSIS RATES

By the late 1970s the number of new cases of tuberculosis in the United States had plateaued, but by 1984, for many reasons, the number of cases started to rise. At the federal level, tuberculosis cases deemed to be the result of reactivation were not, until the late 1970s, counted as new tuberculosis cases, and this may have hindered recognition of problems that had begun earlier. This definitional change artificially altered the national incidence of tuberculosis and may have obscured a true rise earlier and led to a false sense of security. But because "double-books" were not kept (i.e., the original surveillance method was not continued while the change to the new method was occurring), earlier detection of a true rise in incidence was masked. Although some surveillance errors did occur, the magnitude of uncertainty was probably not substantial, however. Whatever the impact of this administrative change, by the mid-1980s the increase in tuberculosis rates was clear at the national level. It has been estimated that between 1985 and 1991 an excess of 39,000 cases was observed nationally above what would have been expected if the downward trend of tuberculosis incidence had continued.[2]

In New York the national trend was amplified. Tuberculosis incidence rates, although they fell in the 1970s, increased steadily in the 1980s (from 19.9 to 36 per 100,000 population between 1980 and 1989), reflecting an average annual increase of 4.4 percent.[3] Even in the 1970s and 1980s pockets of New York City had continued to have substantial rates of tuberculosis. For example, in Harlem between 1969 and 1989, rates of tuberculosis below 100 per 100,000 population occurred in only seven years despite the fact that rates for the United States as a whole steadily fell from just under 20 per 100,000 to under 10 per 100,000.[4] (See figure 3.1.) It is unclear whether inadequacies in local surveillance meant that even these relatively lean years might have been underestimates. What was clear was that in the 1980s New York City had a substantial tuberculosis problem—and the causes were multiple, and many were unknown at the time.

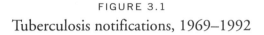

FIGURE 3.1

Tuberculosis notifications, 1969–1992

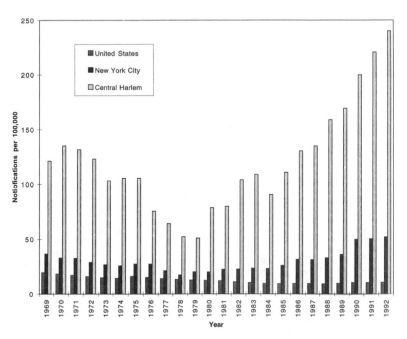

Source: Bureau of Tuberculosis Control, New York City Department of Health; Information Summary 1996.

Undoubtedly the interplay between HIV and *M. tuberculosis* contributed significantly to the resurgence of tuberculosis in the city. The connection between HIV infection and tuberculosis had been first noted in the mid-1980s.[5] By 1988 approximately half of individuals with tuberculosis were also HIV seropositive, and this was reflected in hospital admissions.[6] By 1990 nearly half of all tuberculosis hospitalizations were in patients coinfected with HIV. (See figure 3.2.) AIDS and HIV served to highlight the failures of the public health, welfare, and medical systems, and as HIV prevalence increased, so too did HIV-associated tuberculosis.

HIV in prisoners played an important role in the city's epidemic, a factor more important in New York than elsewhere. By the end of 1988,

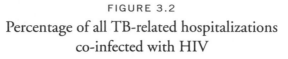

FIGURE 3.2

Percentage of all TB-related hospitalizations co-infected with HIV

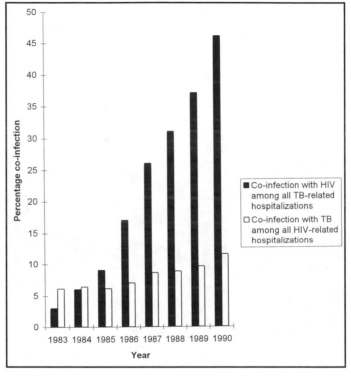

Source: Arno, P. S., et al, "The Economic Impact of Tuberculosis in Hospital in New York City: A Preliminary Analysis," *Journal of Law, Medicine & Ethics* 21 (3-4)(1993): 317-23. Copyright 1993. Reprinted with the permission of the American Society of Law, Medicine & Ethics, Karen A. Bonuck, and Peter S. Arno.

40 percent of all cumulative AIDS cases reported from state correctional systems were reported from New York. This represented 1 percent of all cases of AIDS in the United States. Ninety-five percent of cases had been injecting drug users.[7] More than half of prisoners with tuberculosis were *known* to be HIV infected. (None was known to be HIV seronegative.)[8] Ominously, correlating with the wider problems of drug resistance outside prisons, there were problems with treatment compliance. For example, on Rikers Island, the city's largest and most overcrowded

prison, one study showed that average compliance with chemoprophy-laxis was only 37.5 percent.[9] An expanding inmate population (mark-edly so since the 1970s), crowded living conditions, and the HIV epidemic obviously increased the potential for the spread of tuberculosis in prisons.

Whether the Bureau of Tuberculosis Control was aware of the magnitude of the HIV/tuberculosis problem is uncertain. The first mention of HIV as a cause for concern appears in a 1987 letter by Health Commissioner Stephen Joseph that prefaced the delayed 1984-1985 annual report. The annual reports themselves emphasize HIV only in 1991, when 82 cases of nosocomially acquired (i.e., acquired in hospital) multidrug-resistant tuberculosis were noted. Of these 82 cases, at least 85 percent of patients were coinfected with HIV. Although the annual reports had noted year on year the increases of tuberculosis in the 25- to 44-year age groups and expressed concern "because these are the individuals of child rearing age," the realization that HIV was an important co-factor in the increase in tuberculosis rates took some time. By 1991 tuberculosis incidence rates among black males in the 35- to 44-year age group, for example, were a staggering 469.7 per 100,000, almost 45 times the national average.[10]

The few data available for the homeless population suggest extremely high rates of tuberculosis as well. In studying three New York single-room occupancy (SRO) hotels in the 1970s, Philip Brickner and his colleagues from the Department of Community Medicine at St. Vincent's Hospital found that 6.7 percent had active untreated tuberculosis (more than 300 times the national average).[11] In the mid-1980s active tuberculosis rates in the homeless were calculated at 968 per 100,000 population, compared with a rate of 23 per 100,000 for the New York City population as a whole.[12] At a New York City men's shelter, tuberculosis screening between 1982 and 1988 revealed that 6 percent of men had active tuberculosis and 42.8 percent were found to be infected. By 1992 it was estimated that up to 25 percent of the city's cases of tuberculosis were occurring in the homeless population.[13] Tuberculosis was most common among nonwhite, intravenous drug users, and those who were likely to have spent a considerable number of months living in shelters. Furthermore, the risks of tuberculosis increased with the duration of stay in the shelter system. Completion-of-treatment rates in this population were very low.[14]

The demographic features of tuberculosis patients in Harlem, during a nine-month period in 1988, highlight the characteristics of a population at risk. More than 50 percent of individuals were alcoholic, less than 33 percent were in stable housing, 40 percent had AIDS, and more than 50 percent were intravenous drug users.[15] Perhaps not surprisingly, tuberculosis rates in other deprived populations had increased dramatically over this same period. For example, in the New York State prison population the incidence of tuberculosis increased sevenfold in ten years, from 15.4 per 100,000 in the period from 1976 to 1978 to 105.5 per 100,000 in 1986, and more than 150 per 100,000 in 1991.

Two simple measures indicate a failing control program. The first is tuberculosis incidence in children, because these cases clearly result from recent acquisition rather than reactivation. The second is drug resistance. In New York City between 1987 and 1990, cases in children under 15 years of age rose by 97 percent, from 74 cases to 146. Ninety-two percent of these cases occurred in children aged 4 years or younger.[16] Increasing numbers of very young children were being exposed to *M. tuberculosis,* and active disease was being increasingly seen, especially in blacks. In the Bronx a 300 percent increase in tuberculosis infection rates was seen in preschool children between 1980 and 1992.[17] Overcrowding was the most important contributory factor.

Failing control programs promote the development of drug resistance. Drug resistance in patients who have not been treated previously, which is called primary resistance, is indicative of failures in the past or failures in programs from where individuals have emigrated. When seen in those who have been treated before for a fully susceptible strain (this is known as acquired resistance), contemporary control ("home-grown") program failings are the cause.

Towards the end of the 1980s a substantial rise in drug-resistant tuberculosis cases occurred in New York City. The percentage of cases resistant to at least one drug rose from 19 percent in 1987 to 28 percent in 1991, while resistance to at least both isoniazid and rifampin (i.e., MDRTB) rose from 6 percent to 14 percent.[18] The greatest increases were seen in Manhattan, the Bronx, and Queens. In support of these data, an earlier report had shown that, of isolates (i.e., cultures of tuberculosis from patients) examined during the month of April 1991, 33 percent of tuberculosis cases had organisms resistant to at least one antituberculosis drug, and 19 percent had MDRTB.[19] Furthermore, most multidrug resistance was acquired. (Eighty-one percent of cases with MDRTB had previously received antituberculosis treatment.) Moreover, there had been a significant increase in primary resistance, with rates of resistance to any drug increasing from 10 percent in the 1982 to 1984 period to 23 percent in 1991. In the first quarter of 1991, New York City patients accounted for 61.4 percent of the nation's multidrug-resistant tuberculosis cases.[20]

However, although worryingly high rates of tuberculosis, including drug-resistant tuberculosis, in the homeless had been reported even as late as 1991 the city's Department of Health seems unsure of the magnitude of the drug-resistance problem.[21] The high rate of tuberculosis in the homeless was attributed to the transient lifestyle and social problems of the homeless.[22] In the end the increase in MDRTB was what encouraged public health officials to sit up and take note. High rates of MDRTB brought the existence of nosocomial spread to the attention of those public health officials responsible for the surveillance of patterns of spread. This may not have been obvious if the isolates had been fully sensitive (and therefore not clearly related). In other words, nosocomial spread was recognized because these strains were unusual and could be linked to others epidemiologically. In effect, one failing, that of poor measures to ensure compliance, highlighted a second failing, that of poor infection control in institutions where overcrowding occurred. Indeed, as has been suggested, "We have, in a way, to be thankful for outbreaks of MDRTB for highlighting the problem."[23]

Those living in congregate settings had long been known to be at risk of tuberculosis. As far back as the 1960s it was recognized that New York City prisons were potential reservoirs of tuberculosis.[24] Outbreaks of MDRTB in hospitals and prisons were recognized in the early 1990s.[25] These outbreaks had largely, but not exclusively, involved HIV-infected patients and healthcare workers, with mortality rates of 80 to 90 percent, and with death occurring about one to four months after disease onset.[26] During 1990-1991 in New York State prisons, 171 inmates were diagnosed with tuberculosis, a rate of 156.2 per 100,000. Thirty-nine inmates were found to have epidemiologically linked MDRTB, of whom 38 (97 percent) were coinfected with HIV.[27] In other outbreaks prison guards and healthcare workers uninfected with HIV acquired MDRTB.[28]

Nosocomial spread of tuberculosis, particularly MDRTB, played a major part in the New York City epidemic. This was linked to the high prevalence of HIV-infected individuals in congregate settings and the short incubation period that occurs with HIV-associated tuberculosis. In retrospect, New York City isolates collected between January 1990 and August 1993 have shown that more than one-third of all MDRTB cases had identical or nearly identical molecular patterns, suggesting that they originated from the same strain. Furthermore, the clustered cases in this outbreak, which involved 11 hospitals, represented nearly a quarter of patients with MDRTB in the United States over the period studied. At least 86 percent of patients were HIV infected.[29] A further study that analyzed the molecular epidemiological links of tuberculosis isolates dating from April 1991 showed that, of 344 patients, 126 (37 percent) belonged to one of 31 clusters, and clustering was more frequent in those with MDRTB (involved in 53 percent of clusters), those who were black (44 percent), and those who were homeless (49 percent). A history of incarceration also increased the risk of clustering (although not by a statistically significant amount).[30] Had the study focused on a longer period, it is likely the number of individuals linked to clusters would have been greater. Although spread of MDRTB within congregate settings highlighted failings in infection control, obviously spread of tuberculosis strains fully sensitive to all first-line drugs had also been occurring.

Many who had sought refuge and medical assistance for problems other than tuberculosis, those in shelters and hospitals, for example, had unwittingly exposed themselves to tuberculosis. Others in prisons and jails should have been offered protection were similarly exposed. Many died prematurely. In HIV seropositive individuals, multidrug-resistant tuberculosis is associated with devastating consequences. For example, among 62 HIV-seropositive patients, the median survival was only 2.1 months in one study compared to 14.6 months for controls with tuberculosis caused by single drug-resistant or fully sensitive bacilli.[31] In another study, patients with AIDS and multidrug-resistant tuberculosis were 1.7 times more likely to die than those with drug-susceptible organisms. Ninety-one percent of AIDS patients infected with organisms resistant to both isoniazid and rifampin died with a median survival of about three months.[32]

By 1990 the outlook was bleak. New York City, with 3 percent of the country's population, was accounting for 15 percent of the country's cases. Its incidence rate was five times the national average. It has been estimated that between 1979 and 1994, more than 20,000 cases of tuberculosis occurred in the city above what would have been predicted had the downward trend of the twentieth century continued.[33] But more ominously New York was accounting for more than half of the country's MDRTB cases, the vast bulk of it "home-grown." Numerous outbreaks had occurred in hospitals and prisons and among the homeless. How had this appalling state been arrived at? Three areas require exploration here. The first is the provision of healthcare, both public health and broad medical care; the second is the social transformation that was occurring in New York City that abetted tuberculosis transmission; and third are the social factors that influenced behavior in response to the epidemic, particularly noncompliance. All are intimately related to the development of the epidemic and largely determined the response to it.

HEALTHCARE FAILURES

PUBLIC HEALTH

New York City suffered major economic problems in the early 1970s that culminated, in 1975, in a fiscal crisis. Funding at federal, state, and city levels for tuberculosis programs were slashed. Between 1970 and 1980 national funding fell by 70 percent in real terms, from $40 million to $25 million. Between 1974 and 1980 federal support in the form of Public Health Service funding fell from $1.4 million to $283,000.[34] New York State stopped funding the city's tuberculosis control program entirely in 1979; previously the state's funding had accounted for 50 percent of the support the city had received.[35]

Most public health officials had, up until the late 1980s, believed that transient increases of drug-resistant cases, in particular, were due to immigrants.[36] National surveillance procedures had concentrated on incident rates, or rate of occurrence of the disease, and failed to document prevalence (i.e., the number of cases present at any given time) and, in particular, failure of treatment completion. (In most countries tuberculosis prevalence is still not measured.) Failures in completion of treatment meant that those who had disease had it for a longer time period and prevalence increased out of proportion to increases in incidence. Dr. Eran Bellin of Montefiore Hospital summarized the public health failures in a 1994 editorial in the *Journal of the American Medical Association* (JAMA) in response to a paper describing the magnitude of the New York epidemic: "Our new TB problem is not the result of the United States population's being victimized by infected foreigners, but rather it is the direct result of our society's failure to provide for and then monitor the care of our own citizens."[37]

During the 1970s and 1980s patient care had moved away from being inpatient based in sanatoriums and hospitals to community-based care, as recommended by the 1968 special task force appointed by Mayor John Lindsay.[38] Since 1960 almost all of the 1,000 beds designated for tuberculosis patients had been lost.[39] Yet, as had occurred in mental healthcare provision, no organized community-based model had been set up to respond to the shift to outpatient-based care. The shift from the public (almost all tuberculosis beds were in municipal hospitals) to the private sector (by the late 1970s more than half of all tuberculosis cases were being diagnosed in the private sector) was often inappropriate for patients who, by and large, did not have health insurance and were perceived as being a potential drain on resources.[40] None of the outpatient services that had been recommended by the 1968 task force, including more patient-oriented clinic hours, domicilary and chronic care facilities, and integration of services with care for drug addicts and alcoholics, had been created. In fact, the number of health department chest clinics had been reduced from twenty-two to nine, and none of the suggested improvements in coordination had occurred.

By 1992 problems of leadership in the Bureau of Tuberculosis Control had made matters worse. Clinic physicians were left unsupervised and staff felt unsupported, little attention was paid to patients with MDRTB, and coordination between outreach services and clinic staff was all but nonexistent. Indeed, those patients who were most chaotic were often not brought to the clinic by outreach workers, not because they could not be found, but because workers were concerned about the reception they would receive for bringing an "extra" patient in late in the day. Emphasis was placed on surveillance, not on clinical services, and on the whole, clinics developed autonomously. The director, who was nominally responsible for medical supervision, "hardly ever visited the chest clinics." One staff member, who wishes to remain anonymous, said the director had a "blind trust in the physicians," many of whom were not performing competently. Even with the best will in the world, because of communication failures between clinics and the bureau, many physicians had little information on which to act. For example, when close friends and family members of patients with MDRTB were examined to see if they too were infected, it was often unclear what the correct treatment should be. Those exposed to tuberculosis were frequently simply treated routinely, with inappropriate preventive treatment being offered and inadequate follow-up arranged.

Poor training and supervision of staff, particularly in the shelter system, made matters worse. Karen Brudney and Jay Dobkin of Columbia University, in their comparison of the tuberculosis control programs of New York City and Managua, Nicaragua, commented that public health advisors in New York City (numbering about ten), whose job it was to track down patients in the shelter system, often assumed that a few days treatment each month, when the patients could be located, was better than no treatment.[41] By early 1991 there were only four workers covering 23 shelters.[42] In effect, poor chaotic patients, who should have been a high priority, ended up neglected and received little treatment, rather than complete treatment or no treatment, the worst of all possible scenarios. Among other factors, HIV, overcrowding, inhumane shelters for the homeless, and poor infection control in prisons, hospitals, and other congregate settings fanned the embers of drug resistance caused by inadequate healthcare provision.

By 1989 only 60 percent of patients with tuberculosis were completing treatment in New York City; in some locales that figure approached 90 percent.[43] In a Harlem study more than half of the patients, after leaving hospital, never arrived at their first clinic appointment, and within 12 months of discharge 27 percent were readmitted with tuberculosis again. They were then, once more lost to follow-up on discharge.[44]

Attempts to improve treatment completion rates and compliance, including a federally funded Supervised Treatment Program (STP) initiated in 1979 that had shown some promise (increasing treatment completion rates of those enrolled to 95 percent), fell by the wayside because of inadequate financial support. Even in this apparently successful program, however, although treatment completion rates of those enrolled was high, location of many patients was problematic to say the least. During 1984 and 1985, of 305 patients referred for supervision, only 114 (37 percent) were located and enrolled, and by 1987, of the 173 patients identified as appropriate candidates for STP, only 61 were enrolled because of a lack of staff.[45] The homeless were excluded from the program because, for inclusion, patients needed a permanent residence.[46] Even though these programs offered some benefit, they neglected the most needy and were too small to make any substantial impact. By 1989 this fledgling program employed only six workers.[47]

Although the failings of the public health service through the 1970s and 1980s were perhaps the most significant and certainly most easily correlated cause of the rising tuberculosis burden, another factor of perhaps greater importance also played a role: the paucity of medical care available to the uninsured and the poor.

MEDICAL CARE

There is no universal, national healthcare in the United States. Access to healthcare was, and still is, largely dependent on employer-provided health insurance, and persons who are low paid and unemployed often are uninsured.[48] Moreover, on becoming unemployed, few who previously had coverage manage to continue to make the contributions necessary to maintain their health insurance.[49] In 1976, 23 million Americans had no health insurance. By 1990 this figure had risen to 35.7 million nonelderly Americans, or 16.6 percent of the under 65-year-old population; minority groups and those with chronic illnesses were overrepresented among the uninsured.[50] Those with tuberculosis are likely to be uninsured.[51] The uninsured tend to delay seeking healthcare, and their healthcare provision is patchy and focused on emergency rooms, outpatient clinics, and publicly funded health centers. In the early 1980s, in order to avoid footing costly bills, some New York hospitals relocated emergency rooms to neighborhoods where the uninsured, including those with tuberculosis, were less likely to seek care, or they reduced the services offered within established emergency facilities.[52] Public hospitals have reluctantly borne the brunt of the fiscal pressure caused by the increasing number of uninsured persons.

What determines access to healthcare for poor adults in the United States? Most Americans have private health insurance, which they obtain through their employer or the employer of a family member. But during the 1980s, as costs rose, more and more businesses (particularly small ones) stopped offering health insurance.[53] Between 1980 and 1988, for example, the number of individuals covered by private insurance fell by 5 million.[54] Those not covered by private insurance were supported by a variety of other healthcare coverage options, principally Medicare (for the elderly) and Medicaid (for the poor). To people who are not American natives, and for those from Europe in particular, the U.S. healthcare system is bewilderingly complex. Eligibility for care is dependent on many factors, including income, employer, family structure, type of insurance, stage of disease, and area of residence. The following brief summary attempts to illuminate some of the complexity as it applies to an individual with tuberculosis.

In 1965 the Medicaid program was enacted to provide public insurance coverage for *selected* groups of poor people. It is an open-ended entitlement program under which states pay for medical care services on behalf of eligible beneficiaries, and the federal government matches state spending. In essence, Medicaid eligibility has been linked closely to eligibility for welfare assistance (although this link widened in the late 1980s and has widened further with the recent welfare reform). One-parent families with children, the elderly (who are also covered by Medicare), and the disabled are covered. Up until the recent welfare reform of the late 1990s states were required to extend Medicaid coverage to all recipients who received Aid for Families with Dependent Children (AFDC), namely single-parent families, usually mothers, and to most elderly and disabled people who receive cash assistance from the Supplemental Security Income (SSI) program. Coverage of unemployed two-parent families, children up to age 18 from low-income families, and medically needy families whose incomes are within 133 percent of the income standard for AFDC is optional for states. There is, therefore, variability between states regarding who is eligible for Medicaid. Many states do not extend coverage to two-parent families or to medically needy individuals who are impoverished by large medical expenses, and many poor families are not covered because state income standards for AFDC and Medicaid eligibility fall too far below the poverty level. In addition, the services covered by Medicaid vary among states, with many states imposing limits on the number of hospital days or physician visits covered in a year.[55] In summary, therefore, Medicaid fails to cover all poor people, and in particular those in low-paid jobs without employer-based health insurance, and fails to provide comprehensive benefits to those who are eligible.

During the 1980s several changes were made to the Medicaid program. Some of these were attempts by the federal government to reduce expenditures and others expanded coverage, for example, covering poor pregnant women and children (with poverty being federally determined rather than set at state level). Coverage was extended to *eligible* homeless people—that is, those in poor families with children, pregnant women, and so on, but not all homeless people.[56] Partly as a consequence of these changes, in New York City the number of people eligible for Medicaid increased from 1,194,293 in 1980 to 1,724,018 in 1992. But healthcare coverage for men and childless women was, and continues to be, conspicuous by its absence. These "undeserving" individuals are not eligible.

Despite the expansion of federal-state programs, many people fell through the cracks in the healthcare system, either because they were ineligible for Medicaid or they did not receive employer-provided insurance. Most received their care, as noted earlier, in hospital emergency rooms, outpatient clinics, and publicly funded health centers. In the 1980s, with financial cutbacks occurring at a time when the number of uninsured was increasing in New York, emergency rooms became more crowded, public health centers closed, fewer primary care physicians could be persuaded to work in those that remained, and follow-up of uninsured patients became erratic at best and nonexistent in many cases.[57]

In the 1980s and early 1990s a patient with tuberculosis in New York might well have been uninsured (approximately 25 percent of current tuberculosis cases are eligible for Medicaid) but upon admission to a hospital he or she would have become eligible for emergency Medicaid.[58] This insurance, however, would have ceased on discharge, but care would continue for free through overcrowded state- and city-funded public clinics. If, however, tuberculosis was not suspected—say the diagnosis was a simple bacterial pneumonia—the patient would, on discharge, receive a bill from the hospital. Although the hospital administration may have been aware that the patient was unable to pay, the bill would be issued anyway so the hospital could be reimbursed for the cost of the patient care from the state's "bad debt pool." The patient would, of course, not know this. He or she would continue to receive bills, become increasingly anxious over the possibility of appalling indebtedness, and presumably delay seeking care at a later date.[59]

The uninsured, not surprisingly, use fewer services, receive less inpatient and ambulatory care, and are treated differently when they do receive care.[60] This differential in care provision has translated, again not too surprisingly, in poorer health outcomes for those unprovided for, particularly minority groups.[61] Inpatient mortality rates are higher for the uninsured.[62] Infant mortality rates in the United States, although falling, have failed to decline to the degree seen in other developed nations, and this has been shown to be directly related to poor health coverage for the poor.[63] The risk of death in pregnancy in New York City is four times higher among blacks than whites and in part is related to lack of medical insurance.[64] In 1990 a study of mortality in Harlem found that death rates were higher at most ages after infancy than they were in rural Bangladesh; Harlem had the highest number of drug deaths in the country and also disproportionately high mortality rates from homicide, alcohol, and cirrhosis of the liver.[65] These facts obviously reflect not simply inadequate healthcare provision but also wider social ills.

In summary, although the healthcare system in the United States costs substantially more than any other industrialized nation, it is extremely fragmented and fails to provide good care for those most in need.[66] In 1987 Uwe Rheinhardt, Professor of Political Economy at Princeton University, argued that "Americans spend about three percent of their GNP [gross national product] for the luxury of not having national health insurance."[67] This figure has increased over time. The system nominally gives some Americans greater choice (at the expense of offering others limited care) and any apparent threat to "choice," however restricted that choice may have become, is resisted. Incremental change, which is today accepted as the only politically acceptable way forward, means that this inequitable distribution of healthcare services undoubtedly will continue, despite a popular wish for broader healthcare provision as witnessed by poll after poll in the early 1990s. In 1990 Max Michael, medical director of Birmingham Health Care for the Homeless, bluntly summed up the frustratingly incremental political nature of healthcare system reform both broadly and with regard to the homeless in his contribution to the book *Under the Safety Net:*

The institutionalization of chaos means that those who are responsible for national health policy—namely, the U.S. Congress, the medical profession, state and local governments, consulting firms, to name a few—expend enormous amount of time and energy tinkering with a grossly inadequate system. Each seemingly genuine effort to improve access to care disturbs the healthcare system elsewhere, requiring additional effort to preserve it and the paradigm. The currently fashionable and necessarily transient interest in healthcare for the homeless is an example of the consequences of policy initiatives within the existing paradigm.[68]

THE SOCIAL TRANSFORMATION OF NEW YORK CITY

Most large cities in the United States underwent a transformation in the 1980s. With regard to tuberculosis, the changes had two important effects. First, the increased overcrowding, homelessness, and spread of HIV improved the environmental conditions on which the transmission of tuberculosis thrives. Second, the alienation of a substantial minority of the urban population, in association with the fractured healthcare system, meant that encouraging compliance with treatment over a prolonged period became increasingly difficult.

During the 1980s the dominant image of the underclass became one of individuals with serious character flaws who had only themselves to blame for their social problems. This concept of "blaming the victim" has a long history touched on elsewhere in this book. As Karen Brudney has suggested in regard to tuberculosis and society's most vulnerable, "the basic inability and/or willful refusal to regard this population as coming from the same tribe as the rest of us continue[d] to warp and distort the analyses and solutions offered up by the public sector."[69] It is clear, therefore, that to understand the public health response to the epidemic, one must understand, in addition to the epidemiology and the healthcare failings, the social context in which the seeds of the epidemic were sown. Only by illuminating the social ills and the policies that, in large part, allowed the seeds of tuberculosis to germinate and flourish can the tuberculosis resurgence, the public health response, and, in particular, the use of detention as part of that response be fully understood.

OVERCROWDING

Homelessness and overcrowding increase an individual's risk of exposure to tuberculosis and consequently the risk of active tuberculosis is greater among those living under these conditions. In addition, compliance becomes more of a problem for the homeless because other more urgent practical issues assume greater importance, such as food and shelter.[70] During the 1980s overcrowding in New York City increased. Census data for 1980 and 1990 show that in the Bronx, for example, households having more than one person per room increased from 11.5 percent to 17.5 percent.[71] This overcrowding resulted in part from reductions in municipal services in the 1970s, especially fire control, in poor areas of high population density, which resulted in destruction of housing by fire and the abandonment of buildings. Between 1969 and 1976, for example, 35 firefighting companies were removed, 27 of which had served poor neighborhoods.[72] The cuts in fire service led to an epidemic of building fires in poor areas, with late and inadequate firefighting responses.[73] And increased overcrowding caused further fires. This led to the type of devastation made familiar to those living in the United Kingdom by the BBC documentary, *The Bronx Is Burning.*

Compounding the reduction of fire services, disinvestment in housing, particularly from the private sector, led to further abandonment, which peaked during the city's fiscal crisis of the 1970s. This was most noticeable in inner city neighborhoods such as Central and East Harlem; the Lower East Side in Manhattan; Bushwick, Brownsville, Bedford-Stuyvesant, and East York in Brooklyn; South Jamaica in Queens; and the South Bronx.[74] In Harlem, for example, by the early 1980s one-quarter of residential properties had been abandoned.[75] Aggravating this loss of available housing, federal expenditure, through Community Development Block Grants, Neighborhood Self-Help Development grants, subsidies for public housing, and funds for modernizing public housing were all cut back. Between 1980 and 1990 federal expenditure on housing fell by 77 percent (during this period expenditure on the military rose by 46 percent).[76] A Department of Housing and Urban Development (HUD) deputy assistant secretary, in 1985, gave a particularly revealing explanation for this decline in federal funding for social policy: "We're basically backing out of the business of housing, period."[77]

Gentrification, particularly in inner city areas bordering more affluent neighborhoods, occurred on a sizable scale through the 1980s. Between 1981 and 1986, 205,000 housing units in New York City were converted, most of them to more expensive residencies. Further displacement of the poor was the consequence.[78] New housing was directed predominantly to the wealthier sections of the population. In Manhattan between 1980 and 1987, almost all the 35,000 new housing units authorized were luxury homes.[79]

In New York City, although the loss of housing in the mid-1970s was partly offset by the emigration of 1,393,000 predominantly white, middle-class New Yorkers, 176,000 blacks, 204,000 Hispanics, and 190,000 people of other origins moved into the city. Between 1970 and 1980 the minority population of New York City grew from 36 to 48 percent.[80] These large demographic shifts further disrupted neighborhood social networks. When the emigration stopped, in the late 1970s and early 1980s, and homes were no longer vacated, overcrowding increased.

Overcrowding, therefore, occurred predominantly in the poorer neighborhoods and was directly associated with the rise in tuberculosis incidence. Rodrick and Deborah Wallace, of Columbia University, showed that when the average incidence of new cases of tuberculosis in New York City health districts is plotted against their 1980 "index of extreme housing overcrowding," the linear relationship noted in the early 1970s was transformed into a curvilinear relationship between 1980 and 1985, consistent "with a heightened sensitivity to crowding of a disease in epidemic phase."[81] That is, tuberculosis rates increased, once a threshold had been crossed, out of proportion to the increase in overcrowding. The relationship moved beyond a simple linear one.

HOMELESSNESS

The causes of the increase in homelessness through the 1980s were multifactorial. The most important factors were primarily economic and political, including unemployment, the decline in real wages, problems paying rent, changing family structure, family conflict, declines in the affordability of housing, and population shifts. Deinstitutionalization of the mentally ill in the preceding two decades also significantly contributed to the problem. The 1990 census estimated that in the United

States 230,000 people were homeless, including 180,000 in shelters and 50,000 on the streets. Undoubtedly this was an underestimate. Most conservative estimates put the number of homeless at between 500,000 and 600,000, and others have suggested figures as high as 2 million.[82]

Although the number of homeless individuals is always difficult to deduce reliably, in 1992 it was estimated that 86,000 homeless individuals (or about 1 percent of New York City's population) spent some time in its shelter system.[83] The city's shelter capacity at that time stood at about 9,000 beds, so probably a substantial number of persons spent at least some nights literally on the streets during this period. The stereotypical homeless individual, characterized before the 1970s as a middle-age male alcoholic on skid row, changed during the 1980s when there was an increase in homeless youths, women, families, and the elderly. For example, in one month in 1989 the Human Resources Administration of New York City, in counting the number of individuals housed in shelters and rented hotel rooms, found nearly 4,000 families (including more than 7,000 children).[84]

Just as national deinstitutionalization of the mentally ill had been important in the changing face of the homeless, so too in the case of New York. The scale of deinstitutionalization can be seen if one looks at the decline in the number of inpatients in New York State psychiatric hospitals. In 1955 there were 93,000 psychiatric inpatients. By 1980 this number had declined by 75 percent, to 22,724. By 1992 just over 10,000 patients were inpatients in psychiatric institutions. During the early part of deinstutionalization many mentally ill persons found shelter in SROs, but as reductions in the number of available living units fell, many found themselves without accommodation. Between 1970 and 1982, when the bulk of mentally ill persons were being discharged from psychiatric hospitals, New York lost nearly 90 percent of its SRO stock.[85] Many individuals then drifted from shelters, some to drink and take illicit drugs, and most to go without regular medical or psychiatric care. Many ended up institutionalized again, but this time under the criminal justice system.[86]

In some ways the deinstitutionalization of the mentally ill presented some political groups with a scapegoat. They could describe mental illness as the cause of homelessness. Indeed, President Bush in 1988 made a campaign statement claiming that virtually all the homeless were mentally ill. Although this claim was based on inaccurate estimates, it reinforced the public's perception that "a situation so frightening and unfortunate as homelessness must be caused by mental illness rather than by socioeconomic factors over which people had little control."[87] Despite the exaggerated claims and inferences regarding the association of homelessness and mental illness, the deinstitutionalization of mental hospitals certainly increased the number of mentally ill individuals on the streets, and therefore the proportion of homeless individuals with mental illness increased. More credible evidence suggests that perhaps one-third of the homeless were mentally ill.[88]

Changing family structure during the 1970s and 1980s also contributed to homelessness. During this period young adults were less inclined to live with their parents, the aged lived less with relatives, and children were, more than ever, living in households headed by a single woman. Many of these changes especially affected poor urban blacks. In 1985, for example, 60 percent of black births were to unmarried women compared to 15 percent of white births.[89]

Perhaps exemplifying authority's attitude to the homeless around the late 1980s was the response of Mayor David Dinkins (a black Democrat) to the "shantytown" of approximately 300 homeless people that had developed in Central Park in 1989 as a result of the inadequate shelter accommodation in the city. Police in riot gear destroyed their "homes" and forced the homeless to settle elsewhere.[90] The political emphasis was on ridding the city of the visible consequences of its failed policies, not addressing the causes or dealing humanely with the consequences.

Whether in shelters, SROs, on the streets, or in prisons, the risks of tuberculosis for the homeless were significant. Furthermore, without the support they required (such as assistance with travel, food, alcohol- and drug-dependence), their compliance with antituberculosis drugs was bound to be poor, the risks of drug resistance developing substantial, and transmission to their "neighbors" a real threat.

CRIMINAL JUSTICE SYSTEM AND HIV

Earlier in this chapter I described how tuberculosis rates soared in prisons, particularly in association with HIV. Some have suggested that the prisons and jails of America have served a social role in maintaining control of ill-educated urban blacks and that, by incarcerating a sizable proportion of the poor, the Reagan and subsequently the Bush and Clinton administrations have been able to avoid the difficult questions regarding the economic, political, and infrastructural sources of the nation's inequality, inequity, and poverty. This social control, they contend, has been done through the aggressive, and largely ineffective, War on Drugs, which was initiated in 1972 by President Richard Nixon and escalated by Presidents Reagan and Bush. Whether this is the case or not, incarceration rates have increased dramatically in the United States in recent years, and this increase has been largely of those convicted of drug-related offenses. This trend, of incarceration for drug crimes, has meant both longer sentences for drug-related offenses and, since 1989 with the imposition of mandatory minimum sentencing, increasingly long periods of time actually spent incarcerated.[91]

From 1981 to 1991 the U.S. prison population in state and federal prisons increased from 330,000 to 804,000, and federal drug convictions went up 213 percent.[92] In 1980, 25 percent of the federal prison population was incarcerated for drug charges; by 1992 this figure had risen to 58 percent. New York City, moreover, was one of the front lines in the War on Drugs. Over 250,000 drug-related arrests occurred in 1989 in New York City, and at any given time more than 20,000 drug users were incarcerated in the city's jails with an additional 10,000 to 15,000 in state prisons.[93] This war coincided, perhaps not surprisingly, with the lot of the urban minority population falling to a level well below that of its suburban contemporaries.

This dramatic increase in incarceration rates affected blacks disproportionately. Incarceration rates for blacks, particularly urban blacks, was not necessarily due to differences in drug consumption but to the patterns of drug-related arrests. Blacks account for about 15 to 20 percent of drug users in the United States but in urban areas account for 50 to 67 percent of those arrested for drug offenses.[94] In 1989 in New York City blacks and Hispanics accounted for about half of the population but for 92 percent of all those arrested for drug offenses.[95]

Following arrest, rates of imprisonment also followed racial lines.[96] In 1990 the Sentencing Project cited figures showing that at any given time in the prior year, nationally nearly a quarter of all 20- to 29-year-old black males were under some form of criminal justice sanction, in prison or jail, on probation, or on parole.[97] Another study, assessing those in New York State under criminal justice custody in February

1990, showed that penalties for black and Hispanic men were more severe than for white men. Forty-eight percent of minority male offenders were incarcerated in prison or jail, compared to only 18 percent of white offenders. As with the national study, this local study found that on any given day, one in four young black men was under the control of the criminal justice system.[98] In 1992, more than 80 percent of inmates in New York State facilities were black or Hispanic, in contrast to about 15 percent who were white.

In large part, the political and criminal justice emphasis on crack cocaine fueled this racial imbalance. Possession with intent to supply five grams of crack (which is a crime more likely associated with blacks)[99] brings a mandatory minimum sentence of five *years*. Possession with intent to supply five grams of cocaine (a formulation more likely to be sold and consumed by whites) brings, in contrast, a sentence of 10 to 37 *months*.[100] In effect, the minor pharmacological alterations made to cocaine to produce crack results in a minor modification in pharmacological properties but a dramatic modification in the criminal justice response.

The War on Drugs, in addition to increasing incarceration rates and overcrowding in prisons and jails, and providing an economy in the ghettos, had another important effect related to tuberculosis spread and control: It increased the spread of HIV. It was understood early on in the HIV epidemic that the virus could be spread when drug users shared unsterilized needles. HIV could pass to those sharing their "works," to their sexual partners, and consequently to their children (at birth or through breast-feeding). It has been estimated that there are between 170,000 and 200,000 injecting drug users in the city and that between 1978 and 1984 HIV spread rapidly through that population, reaching a seroprevalence of about 50 percent by the mid-1980s.[101] It was not until 1992, however, that the first sizable legal needle exchange program came into being in New York, several years after similar programs had been set up in Europe and more than a decade after AIDS was first described. Of note it was only in 1988, after it became clear that heterosexual transmission from male injecting drug users to their female partners was occurring in the city, that the state allowed the city to start a small needle exchange program. The mayor closed this down after 14 months because of political opposition. Up until the early 1990s, therefore—a decade after the first AIDS cases had been described—the response of state and federal authorities to the potential spread of HIV among drug users in New York and other East Coast cities "can only be characterized as extraordinarily feeble."[102] The reasons for this feebleness of policymakers were the concerns of both liberal and conservative politicians: Conservative politicians were sensitive to the traditional conventional views of their constituents and were morally outraged by the suggestion that needle exchange services should be developed. They believed that needle exchanges would encourage drug use. Some black liberal politicians were also concerned, but for somewhat different reasons—that needle exchanges would encourage drug use and that this might destroy black communities.[103] Indeed, even funding for bleach distribution programs (bleach is an effective viral sterilizing agent) had been cut, because it supposedly condoned drug use and gave "the wrong message," according to Dr. Woodrow Myers, a former health commissioner.[104] Change eventually came, not through political leadership but from the courts.

In 1990 ten activists, working illegally to provide needles and syringes to injecting drug users, were arrested for illegal possession of syringes and drug paraphernalia. In June 1991 they were found "not guilty by public health necessity" in the state court; shortly thereafter, in 1992, needle exchanges were started once again and expanded rapidly. This time they were legal.[105]

Partly because of the early lack of needle exchanges, but also because of aggressive policing methods predating their inception, HIV spread rapidly through the injecting drug-using population. In marginalizing and repressing these people, the War on Drugs has aggravated the spread of HIV. Proportionately more addicts inject in New York City than elsewhere where policies are directed toward controlling the use of drugs rather than the elimination of drugs. For example, in Rotterdam less than 25 percent of opiate addicts inject, compared to more than 90 percent in New York. The precarious availability of drugs and the aggressive policing policies encouraged "shooting galleries" where addicts congregated to use drugs, as occurred in Edinburgh, Scotland, with equally disastrous results in terms of HIV spread as those in New York City. These "galleries" enabled injecting drug users access to more reliable drug sources, in somewhat greater privacy, with friends and acquaintances. But due to shortage of needles, the injection equipment was used over and over again, spreading HIV and other bloodborne pathogens.[106]

In addition to acquisition through injecting, noninjecting drug users, particularly those using crack, had an increased risk of HIV acquisition through sex. This was related to poverty and the use of sex in transactions for either money or drugs. Trading sex for drugs, in particular crack, was related to poverty first and foremost, and it was therefore poverty that played a substantial part in the heterosexual spread of HIV in New York.[107]

The policies of New York City's authorities toward drug users resulted in HIV rates in injecting drug users and heterosexuals who either used drugs or whose partners used drugs escalating to substantially higher levels than seen in European cities with more relaxed, progressive policies. The HIV prevention policy in prisons further increased HIV spread. Very few U.S. correctional facilities had policies allowing the distribution of condoms to male prisoners (homosexuality is still illegal in some states), and there was no distribution system for bleach or clean needles.[108] Even when condoms were distributed, for example, on Rikers Island, it was through healthcare providers, and most inmates felt inhibited in taking them largely because of a fear of being perceived as homosexual. Furthermore, because sexual activity was prohibited, sex was frequently hurried and often nonconsensual increasing the risk of HIV transmission.[109]

Given that approximately a quarter of state prisoners have injected drugs at some time in their lives, and that one and a half million people are imprisoned (in federal, state, and city institutions) on any given day, it is not surprising that the few studies that have been conducted show that high-risk behavior occurs in prisons and that some prisoners enter without HIV infection but leave infected.[110] The criminal justice system has done little to contain the spread of HIV and consequently tuberculosis. In fact, it could be argued, it encouraged the spread of both. The broad public health response to HIV has often been to emphasize the moral virtues of abstinence from both sex and drug use rather than to promote harm reduction.[111]

A postscript to the story of needle exchange suggests that at the federal level, there is still enthusiasm for such moral hand-wringing rather than pragmatic policymaking. In 1998 the Clinton administration, rejecting public health evidence and advice, declined to lift the nine-year ban on federal financing for programs to distribute clean needles to users. This was despite evidence clearly showing that such programs reduce the spread of HIV and also, politically more important, that such programs do not encourage drug abuse. The reason given for maintaining the ban was that lifting it would "send the wrong message to the nation's children." These same sentiments were being expressed more than a decade earlier and beg the question: What *is* the right message to send to children? Beyond the standard war refrain of "Just Say No," messages encouraging compassion, tolerance, and support for the most vulnerable seem lost. Indeed, where the use of illegal drugs is concerned, pragmatic public health promotion, rather than political rhetoric, always seems to come a poor second. Ultimately it was simply political expediency—congressional elections just a few months away— that made Clinton maintain the ban. As of mid-1999, it has been estimated that there are only approximately 100 programs operating nationally, but they remain illegal in many states including several with a large number of injecting drug users and substantial HIV prevalence rates.[112] Thousands of people are continuing to get infected by sharing needles, and children born to mothers with HIV continue to be infected.

Several other factors beyond overcrowding, homelessness, drugs, HIV, and the criminal justice system also expanded the fractures in New York's poor neighborhoods. Although they did not influence tuberculosis transmission directly, they probably made treatment of some patients more problematic.

THE SEEDS OF "RECALCITRANCE"

Some have suggested that the recalcitrant, noncompliant tuberculosis patient in New York had "only himself to blame." This implies that "delinquency" or "recalcitrance" is set at birth, and social influences make little difference to behavior. But this is clearly sheer nonsense. Beyond skepticism that a single gene or group of genes can influence such a varied pattern of behavior, there is overwhelming evidence to support the thesis that the environment plays a substantial part in molding behavior. "Recalcitrance" cannot be viewed simply as the product solely or primarily of individual pathology, ignoring the institutional forces in society that help perpetuate deprivation, marginalization, alienation, and hopelessness. If one accepts that social deprivation can lead to isolation and social exclusion of individuals, I believe one also can assume that these forces actively encourage a sense of futility, hostility, and inevitably a reluctance to cooperate; in other words, "noncompliance." And this noncompliance is not passive but active, an attempt to vent frustration and gain self-esteem.

Follow-up of children from studies begun in the 1970s, for example, clearly show that antisocial behavior is associated with many factors, including genetic predisposition, but also perinatal problems, parenting, poverty, and violent or socially disorganized neighborhoods.[113] Some of these factors, such as low socioeconomic status and poor parenting, weigh more heavily in producing delinquent behavior, while others have a less marked effect. But most of these influences do not work in isolation. For example, poverty potentiates the consequences of perinatal problems, and good parenting reduces the impact of poverty on delinquency. Delinquency, or antisocial behavior, like most human behavior, develops through an interplay of multiple influencing factors, many of them social. And just as adverse social conditions may promote antisocial behavior, so supportive families and communities can improve behavior.[114] Distilling which are the dominant factors in provoking "recalcitrant" behavior is complex, but many of the issues to be discussed probably played, and continue to play, a part.

Further support for the impact society, and particularly inequality or "relative deprivation," plays in influencing behavior can be gleaned from a study from John Johnstone in Chicago. In the late 1970s he found that poor teenagers with wealthy neighbors committed more serious crimes than poor teenagers from poor neighborhoods.[115] This supports the "gut" belief that the sense of futility, hopelessness, and alienation engendered when inequality is associated with lack of opportunity (or equality of life chances) will likely have an effect on delinquency or recalcitrance.[116] Deference to authority, whether it is medical authority or other sources such as police, may be affected. Marked inequality makes the gap between promise and fulfillment more glaring, which may help to explain the behavior of some recalcitrant individuals. This gap has been described metaphorically as the "tunnel effect." When drivers are caught in a traffic jam in a tunnel, they are initially pleased when cars on either side begin to move. But when movement on either side continues yet they do not start to move, they feel that they are in a relatively worse position. Frustration eventually turns to anger and rebellion.[117] Resentment leads to delinquency. This metaphor serves well when one considers the juxtaposition of the "Gordon Geckos" of the 1980s, those displaying their wealth (and greed) ostentatiously (like Michael Douglas's character in the movie *Wall Street*), with those for whom the opportunity of advancement was poor. It was from these poor populations that most "delinquents" came and that those ultimately detained because of poor treatment compliance came.

A further strand of evidence (and there are many others) supporting the belief that environment influences behavior comes from psychologists and psychiatrists.[118] Viktor Frankl, a Jewish psychiatrist, in describing his experiences in a Nazi concentration camp, eloquently addresses this sense of distance from "normal" behavior that ensues under appalling suffering and how one's responses to others are altered in such circumstances. With regard to the frequent beatings he and others suffered, he records: "Apathy, the blunting of the emotions and the feeling that one could not care any more, were the symptoms arising during the second stage of the prisoner's psychological reactions, and which eventually made him insensitive to daily and hourly beatings. By means of this insensibility the prisoner soon surrounded himself with a very necessary protective shell." He later noted, "The most painful part of beatings is the insult which they imply."[119] The more excluded from mainstream American society some individuals become, and the more their sense of injustice increases, the more their behavior will differ from what is accepted as "normal" and moral. In the 1960s, sociologist H. S. Becker suggested that the more a marginalized group is repressed and ostracized, the more it will see itself as a marginalized group, and the more the behavior of group members will be outside the norms and values of the wider society but normal and valued from within the group, therefore reinforcing that "deviant" behavior.[120] In other words, the more prevalent chaotic and destructive behavior is within a community, the more it is accepted and the lower the social costs of the violating "normal" values. During the 1980s communities in many American cities, not least New York City, became severely fractured and accepting of destructive behavior.

The stresses that were felt in the cities were focused on the poor. Many residents in extreme poverty had little social support, fewer social ties, and were more isolated. Many had no partner, some could not claim a "best friend," and marriages were less likely to survive. Individuals were less likely to participate in community organizations and social groups. In sum, the resources they could draw on were fewer, the "social capital" they gained through being socially integrated, less.[121] Other factors compounded this deteriorating situation.

Crack in particular had a devastating impact on these fragile communities. Mindy Fullilove, working from the Community Research Group in New York, described the crack epidemic as "a tsunami, a tidal wave, that swept through neighborhoods in New York in the late eighties, early nineties. It was enormously destructive."[122] Others have attested to this as well. Crack was "like a bullet wound to the communities that were already suffering. Even if the bullet can be safely extracted, it has left these neighborhoods deeply scarred."[123] The effect of crack was, in part, because of the immediacy of the pharmacological response. The dark depression that follows the crack "high" causes an urgency to feed the habit not seen with other illicit drugs. This urgency created a market into which stepped new young dealers, most of whom carried guns, with consequent territorial disputes being settled by violence that further increased many people's sense of isolation.

As I have previously noted fire, like crack, swept through some poor neighborhoods. In destroying buildings it destroyed the social network within communities. Senior citizen groups, political clubs, churches, and youth groups disintegrated. Communities lost their cohesive bonds.[124]

CHANGING EMPLOYMENT TRENDS

One of the most fundamental changes that occurred in inner cities during the 1970s and 1980s, particularly in the North, was a change in the pattern of employment, particularly among black youths. The economic transformation of cities in the postindustrial era meant that the number of jobs requiring a low level of educational attainment fell markedly during those decades. This lack of work opportunity, compounded by poor inner city educational resources, kept many from the primary labor market, a large proportion of them permanently.

There had been a marked expansion of higher education in the United States from the 1950s to the 1970s; in 1945 only one in five Americans received postsecondary education, yet by 1992 four in five did.[125] This access to education undoubtedly helped make America a more equal society. New York State had been in the vanguard of this movement. For those with a college degree, there ceased to be a connection between the occupational status of their parents and their own.[126] Expansion of higher education had led to the expansion of opportunity for many. But some were left behind. Those who did not graduate from college (and even more so those who had failed to complete their high school education) faced a bleak future. During the 1980s the earnings of college graduates rose while the earnings of those who had not attended college fell.[127] The educational attainment of minority males, particularly blacks, and especially in the inner cities, fell well short of that of city-based whites. Whereas most city-based whites attended college, most blacks did not, and many did not complete high school.[128] Some commentators contend that many inner city schools provide a "repressive, arbitrary, generally chaotic internal order, coercive authority structure and minimal possibilities for advancement" that by its nature, influences behavior and alters individual value systems.[129] For whatever reason, inner city minority youths were failing to enjoy the benefits of a college education with dire consequences.

With the manufacturing base dwindling, even individuals who had been steadily employed lost their jobs. Between 1972 and 1982 New York City lost 30 percent of its manufacturing jobs.[130] New jobs for the ill-educated tended to be in the service industries, were low paid and offered little security, and few gave benefits such as health insurance. Many of those who did find work, therefore, remained poor, "because their low wages and occupational immobility trapped them in poverty despite their commitment to the work ethic."[131] In New York City in 1980 nearly 40 percent of black males had not graduated from high school, and more than 50 percent of black men who had failed to graduate from high school were not working, whereas only 4 percent of black males with college qualifications were unemployed.[132] In New York City between 1970 and 1987, although black employment declined by 84,000 in manufacturing industries (where employers require lower levels of education), black employment increased by 104,000 in public administration and professional services (jobs requiring high-level education). So although opportunities for well-educated individuals improved, opportunities for the poorly educated declined markedly during this period.[133]

POVERTY

Social policy analyst Peter Townsend described poverty as "the lack of the resources necessary to permit participation in the activities, customs, and diets commonly approved by society."[134] From this description it is clear that poverty is more than simply a measure of low income. It is a measure of an individual's ability to be involved in society. Throughout the 1970s and 1980s many communities in New York City became more impoverished. Large parts of the city became "extreme poverty neighborhoods" or ghettos. That is, they became areas of concentrated poverty in which, in sociologist William Julius Wilson's definition, at least 40 percent of the people residing within the neighborhood are poor.[135]

Although the poverty threshold often shifts in attempts to mask the scale of poverty for political reasons, it is clear that the number of Americans living below this line increased in the 1980s.[136] For example, between 1979 and 1990 the number of blacks living below the poverty level increased from 18.5 percent to 25.3 percent, and for whites, from 11.4 percent to 17.1 percent.[137] By 1991, 35.7 million people (14.2 percent) were living in poverty, a much higher proportion than in other affluent industrialized nations.[138] By 1990 the "underclass"—that is, those individuals permanently stuck at the bottom of American society—had swollen to three million, most of them minorities residing in large cities.[139]

Between the 1950s and the 1980s the poor became concentrated in the centers of cities in America. For example, between 1959 and 1985 the proportion of poor in these areas grew from 27 percent to 43 percent, and blacks were overrepresented. During the same period the increase in poor blacks in city centers increased from 38 percent to 61 percent. By 1980 almost a third of all metropolitan blacks lived in ghettos; 65 percent of the 2.4 million ghetto poor in the United States were black, 22 percent Hispanic, and 13 percent non-Hispanic and other races.[140] This concentration of poverty affected some cities more than others, but New York was undoubtedly one of those most severely affected. It was one of just four cities that accounted for three-quarters of the growth in city poverty. (The others were Chicago, Philadelphia, and Detroit.)[141] Indeed, one-third of the increase in ghetto poverty in the United States in the 1970s occurred in New York City alone.[142]

With a recession and the shift in ideological thinking under Reagan, city governments across the country cut social services, state governments made savings by introducing more restrictive rules for general assistance (otherwise known as relief), and the federal government cut back on social programs. During their economic travails in the 1970s and 1980s, ordinary Americans and their elected representatives focused on welfare and its beneficiaries.[143] Between the 1970s and 1985 AFDC benefits declined by a third in real terms and general assistance dropped by 32 percent. In addition, thousands of disabled people were removed from the Supplemental Social Security lists. In New York State in 1980, 13.8 percent of individuals were living below the poverty line. By 1992 this figure had risen to 16.4 percent.[144]

INEQUALITY

Income inequality for Americans has become more profound since the mid-1970s. Economists Peter Gottschalk and Timothy Smeeding illustrated the differences in inequality between different nations in the 1980s and early 1990s. (See figure 3.3.) Even allowing for variations in data collection, different time frames, and different methodologies, inequality in the United States was far more profound than elsewhere, with earnings at the bottom lower than in many other countries and earnings of those with high incomes substantially higher than their colleagues elsewhere.[145] Inequality has increased over time when one compares the lowest 20 percent with the top 20 percent in terms of disposable personal income. Between 1977 and 1990 the poorest 20 percent of the population suffered a 15 percent loss in real income, while the wealthiest one-third of the population gained in wealth. (The wealthiest 1 percent increased their after-tax income by 110 percent.)[146] Whereas the richest 20 percent of households' annual income increased by $28,000 in the two decades leading up to 1990, the income of the middle 60 percent increased only by $4,600, and the incomes of the poorest 20 percent of households *fell* by $200 per *person*.[147] Another way of looking at this disparity is to compare the earnings of chief executive officers (CEOs) with their workers'. By 1990 an average American CEO received $120 for every dollar earned by the average worker. (By 1994 this figure had increased to $225.) For comparison, the ratio in Britain around 1990 was 25 to 1, and in Germany 21 to 1.[148]

FIGURE 3.3

Real earnings distribution comparison for full-time full-year males in 1991 United States dollars

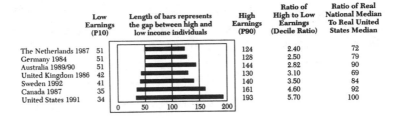

	Low Earnings (P10)	Length of bars represents the gap between high and low income individuals	High Earnings (P90)	Ratio of High to Low Earnings (Decile Ratio)	Ratio of Real National Median To Real United States Median
The Netherlands 1987	51		124	2.40	72
Germany 1984	51		128	2.50	79
Australia 1989/90	51		144	2.82	90
United Kingdom 1986	42		130	3.10	69
Sweden 1992	41		140	3.50	84
Canada 1987	35		161	4.60	92
United States 1991	34		193	5.70	100

Source: P. Gottschalk, and T. M. Smeeding, "Cross-national Comparisons of Earnings and Income Inequality," *Journal of Economic Literature* 35 (June 1997): 633-87. Copyright 1997. Reprinted with the permission of the American Economic Association.

Inequality in America in the 1980s became more pronounced, with the rich becoming richer and the poor becoming poorer.

In New York the disparity was wider than that seen nationally. By the mid-1990s the richest 20 percent of families with children had average incomes 20 times as great as the poorest 20 percent of families. (Nationally, by this time, the richest 20 percent had average incomes approximately 13 times as great as the poorest 20 percent.) Between the late 1970s and the mid-1990s, whereas nationally the average income for the poorest fifth of families fell by $2,500 (from $11,760 to $9,250), in New York the income for the poorest fifth of families fell by $3,800 (from $10,590 to $6,790). In New York, during the same period, the richest fifth of families increased their income by, on average, $41,580 (from $90,810 to $132,390).[149] So New York, as ever, illustrated on a grander scale the poverty, the affluence, and the inequality seen elsewhere.

IDEOLOGICAL SHIFT

During the 1980s the straits of the urban poor in America worsened dramatically. The ideology of the 1960s and 1970s was abandoned during this decade. The Reagan administration broadly rejected "social engineering" (the use of incentives and disincentives to affect human behavior in order to improve conditions) in favor of a greater commitment to individualism and individual economic freedom. In short, the administration rejected governmental control over social policy. The fortieth U.S. President memorably summarized this position when he said at his inauguration in 1981, "Government is not the solution to our problems. Government is the problem." The era of "Big Government" was over. But not quite. During Reagan's presidential tenure the federal deficit grew from $73.8 billion to $155 billion. The era of "Big Government" was not over, it had simply refocused its sights (literally as well as metaphorically). Support for social programs waned as spending on the military increased. The solution to an economic malaise that was, notably, affecting the middle classes was clear. As sociologists Claude Fischer and his colleagues of the University of California succinctly put it in describing the support Reagan enjoyed:

> In the early 1980s, one explanation dominated public discussion and public policy: The cause of the middle-class crisis was government, and its solution was less government. Regulations, taxes, programs for the poor, preferences for minorities, spending on schools—indeed, the very size of government—had wrecked the economy by wasting money and stunting initiative, by rewarding the sluggards and penalizing the talented. The answer was to get government "off the backs" of those who generate economic growth. "Unleash the market" and the result would be a "rising tide that will lift all boats, yachts and rowboats alike."[150]

Libertarian Adam Smith's "invisible hand" would be ungloved.

Shortly after Reagan assumed the presidency, it was clear that there was little concern for the poor or increasing equality, and welfare programs suffered. The Reconciliation Act of 1981 and the budget of 1982 confirmed this ideological shift. The 1982 budget cut expenditures by approximately $30 billion, or 6 percent of baseline expenditure.[151] These cuts, although only a small proportion of the overall budget, were focused most on the poor and their welfare support, rather than on the more politically powerful recipients of Social Security and Medicare. It was felt that special programs for the poor undermined the incentives to work, and political attempts in the preceding years (since the civil rights movements of the mid-1960s) to improve the lot of the poor had, in large part, failed to achieve their goals. But it was also recognized that the recipients of Medicare and Social Security were a potent political force; the poor were not. This ideological shift, which included an increased emphasis on moral behavior, broadly determined social policy throughout the Reagan and Bush presidencies (and continues to do so under President Clinton).

CONCLUSION

The public health system in New York City had failed to detect and act on increasing tuberculosis rates, failed to grasp the causes or understand the implications, and failed to provide for those most in need until 1992. The advice of experts in previous years had been disregarded in a futile effort to save money. Patients had fallen between what were sizable cracks in the system. Furthermore, the fractured medical system, in its bureaucratic tangle, had failed to provide any continuity of care, focusing rather on in-hospital care, particularly for the insured. Policymakers disregarded the threat of communicable diseases to those unable to access long-term care. The social transformation the city underwent during this period compounded the inadequacy of healthcare provision for the poorest. Overcrowding, homelessness, and HIV all combined to provide the perfect milieu for tuberculosis development and transmission.

The inequalities and lack of opportunity for sizable numbers of the urban population led to disenchantment, a sense of futility, and ultimately, in some, hostility. Certainly some individuals were galvanized while experiencing this adversity and, through great effort and ability, succeeded and escaped poverty to enjoy the fruits others in society were enjoying. Others, however, formed alternative subcultural social orders. Some became ever more isolated, resentful, and alienated—the "recalcitrant" few.

Thus tuberculosis, an eminently treatable disease requiring a "low-tech" response, spread to infect many of the most vulnerable, in settings where institutions should have been obliged to offer protection, with devastating consequences. Those who were most affected by the epidemic, and ultimately were the greatest challenge to the control program, originated from the poorest neighborhoods. Most were not actively "delinquent" but had to surmount very high hurdles to access care. A few, however, were truly recalcitrant, truly hostile to authority, and resistant to inducements to comply with therapy. These recalcitrant, delinquent individuals with tuberculosis are the ones New York City authorities sought to control. The city responded to the problem not by reconsidering the institutional and political structures that had caused the mass of urban decay (which they would, in any case, have been largely impotent to change) but by addressing it from a narrow public health perspective, as I shall describe in the next chapter.

When Push Comes to Shove

Many politicians of our time are in the habit of laying it down as a self-evident proposition, that no people ought to be free till they are fit to use their freedom. The maxim is worthy of the fool in the old story, who resolved not to go into the water till he had learnt to swim. If men are to wait for liberty till they become wise and good in slavery, they may indeed wait for ever.

—Thomas Babington Macauley,
Essays Contributed to the Edinburgh Review, 1843

Despite warning signs that parts of New York City had a significant tuberculosis problem years, perhaps even decades, earlier, it was not until the late 1980s that public health officials started to respond in any meaningful way. When, in 1986, Stephen Joseph became commissioner of health, he was made aware of the increasing tuberculosis problem. At that time blame was attributed to the hospitals and physicians who were thought not to be assiduous enough in reporting patients with tuberculosis or responding to their needs.[1] If underreporting was thought to be a problem even when it was known that the situation was deteriorating, one must wonder: How bad was the situation really? As Wafaa El-Sadr, chief of infectious diseases at Harlem Hospital, commented when referring to the tuberculosis situation in 1988 when she started there: "Because the surveillance system had broken down and the system was inadequately funded there was no knowledge of the size of the problem in the first place never mind a plan of what to do."[2] While New York

City, along with other urban centers, was witnessing a major failure in tuberculosis control and, in particular, the rapid expansion of drug-resistant strains, the Centers for Disease Control and Prevention established, on the basis of declining *national* figures for tuberculosis, the Advisory Council for the Elimination of Tuberculosis in 1987. In 1989 a new program announced, with great fanfare, a new program entitled the "Strategic Plan for the Elimination of Tuberculosis in the United States."[3] The irony of the national plan was not lost on those intimately involved with tuberculosis in New York City.

This chapter describes the public health response to the epidemic, detailing the debate regarding the legal response to and the detention of noncompliant, noninfectious individuals. This is not to suggest that other measures initiated were less important, but I believe that it is in this realm that recent changes in the boundaries between liberty, personal responsibility, and state authority are best exemplified. I therefore examine in detail the amendments to the regulations that enabled the city to detain noninfectious individuals (i.e., the regulatory changes that formalized this significant expansion of state authority). A further reason for dissecting this shift in balance is that public health officials viewed the threat of detention as a crucial underpinning of the bureau's efforts to improve treatment completion, reduce drug resistance, and increase its standing among city physicians. This issue is important to examine because other policymakers looking to assert, or reassert, their authority over public health may look to New York for guidance.[4] In order to place in context the regulatory changes, this chapter also briefly describes some measures undertaken to "turn the tide" and outlines the events leading up to these changes.

Several players were involved in these events, including the media, interest groups, health officials and politicians, and I consider their roles and the implications of their responses. As Christopher Foreman, a senior fellow at the Brookings Institution, suggested in his book *Plagues, Products & Politics,* a "primary significance of emergent hazards lies not in the management of the episodes themselves but in the wider and more durable reassessments and reforms they trigger."[5] Only time will tell if this is true of the New York response to tuberculosis, whether the recourse to coercion to ensure compliance persists in the city and elsewhere in the United States, and whether those regions of the world with the resources to enact similar measures will follow New York's lead when (or if) faced with a similar scenario.

MEDIA RESPONSE AND PUBLIC ANXIETY

Several tensions affect policymaking. One is the challenge to provide a workable program that strikes the appropriate balance between urgency and restraint. Another is the degree to which decision making by public health experts can and should be affected by politics. Both of these areas were alluded to by Thomas Frieden when he reflected, six years later, and remembered the following advice given to him by the departing director, Jack Adler: "The art of media relations in TB is the art of controlled hysteria. . . . You want people to be worried enough to give you more resources, but not so worried they make you do all sorts of stupid things."[6] The political process tends to be disordered and unpredictable. Several factors play a part in the development of a response to an emerging public health hazard, and in part because of these tensions, the responses are not always rational.

According to Foreman, health reporters are drawn to four kinds of stories: fire alarms, controversies, human interest, and breakthroughs.[7] The New York City tuberculosis epidemic fulfilled at least the first three of these categories and perhaps the last. Widespread anxiety and fear of potentially untreatable strains of tuberculosis set off alarm bells, and the scandal of the public health failures was standard fare for journalists. The fact that healthcare workers and prison guards were affected added a moral angle and fueled interest with the "undeserving" infecting the "deserving" (or members of the "general public"). The breakthrough news occurred later, with the control of the epidemic, and the public health success was laid at the door of a freshly rediscovered public health response, directly observed therapy.

As was becoming clear in the early 1990s, the critical challenge for public health policy was to ensure that patients complied with their treatment. Multidrug-resistant tuberculosis outbreaks had highlighted the possible consequences of poor compliance in an individual with treatment, particularly among vulnerable persons with AIDS or in congregate settings. The press reports were alarming, sometimes with overt moral overtones. In October 1990 the *New York Post*, for example, ran a headline highlighting the potentially explosive nature of the problem: "TB timebomb. Homeless Contaminate Public Areas in City."[8] The next day, suggesting that all New Yorkers were at risk, the *Post's* front-page headline read: "Highly Contagious Tuberculosis Close to Epidemic Level in the City." The article noted that "No matter where you are in New York today, you can be at risk."[9] Later reports covering the city's tuberculosis problem further increased anxiety. For example, on January 24, 1992, the *New York Times* ran the headline "Deadly Strain of Tuberculosis Is Spreading Fast, US Finds."[10] The following day a headline tempered the previous day's message: "For Most, Risk of Contracting Tuberculosis Is Seen as Small."[11] In a similar vein, the *Smithsonian* reported, again in 1992, the resurgence of tuberculosis with the title "TB: The Disease That Rose from Its Grave."[12]

During the early 1990s the public was increasingly being made aware of the scale of the problem. In concert there arose an ongoing debate in the press about the homeless, illegal drug use, and HIV. Some articles such as a *New York Post's* editorial, "Safeguarding the City against TB," highlighted both the need for isolation ("the goal here is to stop an incredibly dangerous epidemic in its tracks") and civil liberties issues ("[At] some point, the rights of other members of society need to be weighed against the 'right' of TB carriers to take their medicine").[13] Other newspaper articles appeared highlighting the association of tuberculosis among the homeless, the mentally ill, alcoholics, illicit drug users, and public health officials' lack of authority to detain noncompliant patients with tuberculosis. In another editorial entitled "Can Society Protect Itself?" the *New York Post* commented: "These new killer strains are being spread by patients who do not take their TB medicine—leaving the hospital and stopping their medication as soon as their symptoms improve. The city has no enforcement procedures to hold TB patients after they are no longer contagious."[14] Still another editorial in the *Post,* entitled "Dealing with the TB Menace," increased public anxiety further and warned that "while TB may pose a particular danger to people with weakened immune systems—HIV positive men and women, for example—it actually represents an acute public-health threat to *all* New Yorkers."[15] The *New York Times,* in October 1992, ran five consecutive articles on tuberculosis, four of them front-page pieces.[16] The first of these, "Neglected for Years, TB Is Back With Strains That Are Deadlier," quoted Lee Reichman, president of the American Lung Association: "I'm scared. Here we are in 1992 with cure rates lower than countries like Malawi and Nicaragua. We can't keep track of our patients, and all evidence suggests more and more of them have TB that is resistant to our best drugs. We have turned a disease that was completely preventable and curable into one that is neither. We should be ashamed."[17] A New York–based tuberculosis expert, Barry Bloom, commenting on the fragmentation of the healthcare system, said in the same article, "It is hard not to be bitter about a catastrophe that simply should never have happened. We had everything we needed. All the knowledge, the skills, the medical expertise necessary to eliminate this disease. Instead, this country chose to very nearly eliminate the healthcare programs people with this disease need most."[18]

Further adding to the public anxiety and highlighting concerns over personal safety for medical professionals, the October 13 headline of The *New York Times* read "TB, Easily Transmitted, Adds a Peril to Medicine," and Lee Reichman, commenting on nosocomial spread within hospitals, suggested, "All we need is another epidemic, and it will be impossible to staff city hospitals."[19] Perhaps not by coincidence this headline appeared the day before the city's strategic planning meeting was due to take place.[20] One can get a measure of the increasing public interest in tuberculosis during this period, and subsequently, by looking at the number of articles published in general-interest magazines and periodicals. A rapid increase in numbers occurred since 1990. (See figure 4.1.) It is difficult not to conclude that public health officials themselves generated much of the media attention given to the tuberculosis threat. It was public health officials who, as Adler had suggested, used the media to increase anxiety and gain political attention. Many articles were timed to coincide with moves by city officials to gain additional resources— and the peak in media attention actually followed, rather than predated, many of the bureau's changes.

A few years later George Comstock, one America's leading epidemiologists and an authority on tuberculosis, summed up many physicians' attitude to "willfully recalcitrant" patients on public television:

> People who deliberately or carelessly infect other people should be treated like criminals in my opinion. You know, they're just as dangerous as the guy who goes around shooting off a pistol randomly. You know, sooner or later they're going to cause somebody to die with their drug [*sic*]. Just like the guy shooting a pistol randomly sooner or

FIGURE 4.1

Number of articles on tuberculosis according to
Readers' Guide to Periodical Literature

(approximately 250 English language periodicals indexed).

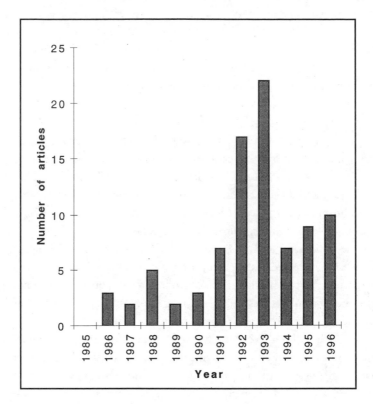

later it's going to kill somebody. And I think we need to have facilities
to put people in hospitals and keep them there until they're cured.[21]

Few media commentators examined the social disintegration that had
helped the epidemic grow or the social policies that had fanned the
flames of the epidemic. Emphasis was largely placed on the underfunding of the public health system, the failure of health systems to respond,
and the abdication of personal responsibility by those infected. This last
group was useful, not least because public ire could be channeled onto
them and, through this, other public health changes enacted. Although

only a small minority of persons with tuberculosis, these recalcitrant few received an inordinate amount of local attention.

POLITICAL RESPONSE

In his March 1987 letter prefacing the delayed 1984-1985 "Tuberculosis in New York City" Report, Stephen Joseph, commissioner of health, pointed out the concern of health officials to the "possible association between tuberculosis and the Human Immunodeficiency, or AIDS, Virus" and the increases in "homelessness and congregate shelter living."[22] By 1987 public health officials tentatively recognized the link of tuberculosis with HIV and Dixie Snider, head of CDC's tuberculosis division, was asked to review the New York tuberculosis program. (Others have suggested that the CDC itself suggested it review this program, and the city's formal request came only after the CDC prompt.) The report from Snider that followed in late 1987 was scathing in its criticism of the city's tuberculosis program. It made several recommendations, including the streamlining of the administration of the Bureau of Tuberculosis Control, the recruitment of new leadership, a clarification of the role of the Department of Health Chest Clinics, an improvement in surveillance, and the development of a citywide comprehensive plan for tuberculosis control.[23] In addition, the report suggested that a long-term care facility for noncompliant patients should be developed. Thus, part of the suggested response was to resurrect the use of coercive measures, which had largely fallen by the wayside, to support broader public health measures. At this time there were no dedicated detention beds in New York, no well-organized DOT programs, and no legal framework to effectively detain individuals once they were no longer infectious.

Joseph later noted that "[p]ublic concern regarding the 'threat' of tuberculosis among the homeless ('threat' in the sense of spread to non-homeless individuals and of possible explosive shelter outbreaks) was very high in 1988–89."[24] When one views the political and media response to the homeless during the 1980s, it could be argued that this might have been rephrased as public concern that the threat *from* the homeless was high. The pressure to respond was great, and Joseph acted by increasing screening, particularly among the homeless. In 1988 a dedicated shelter for homeless tuberculosis patients with voluntary admission and on-site supervised therapy was set up adjacent to Bellevue

Hospital. Joseph also set up and instructed an Expert Advisory Committee to produce a strategic plan, reported later that year.[25] This committee, like Snider's, made several recommendations, including that the DOH institute a laboratory training and support program for hospitals. However, "because of budget constraints, and in part because we did not at the time recognize the far-reaching importance of that recommendation, little was done."[26]

The leadership in the Bureau of Tuberculosis Control, as Snider had noted, was poor. The staff had accepted the inexorable rise in the number of cases yet were unable to respond in any coordinated fashion. Adler, the bureau's part-time director, was frequently not around. Indeed, as time went by, his office was used more and more for staff meetings and conferences (something that caused raised eyebrows after he left). Those intimately aware of the problems, in the chest clinics for example, felt unsupported. Indeed, although they provided care for many uninsured patients, until 1985 they were not under the bureau's direct supervision. But even after 1985 senior public health officials from the bureau rarely visited, and when they did they expressed mild surprise at how busy the staff was. In some areas emphasis was placed on schemes that had little impact but overburdened the already overstretched clinic staff. Frieden recalled some of the problems: "They made some colossal mistakes. In the midst of a ten percent completion rate they mandated that 100,000 school kids had to get a tuberculin test every year. And the reason they did that, if you read the internal documents, was because they wanted everyone to be worried about TB. But it devastated the clinic because it swamped them with nonsense."[27] It took four years for this decision to be reversed.

"Little was done," therefore, despite two expert advisory committees warning of problems ahead. Toward the end of 1991 Margaret Hamburg was made health commissioner by Mayor David Dinkins. Leadership within the bureau also changed. A reluctant Paula Fujiwara was encouraged to start early by the CDC, before a formal change of director had been made. Frieden, who had been based in the clinics as an Epidemic Intelligence Service officer (EIS) from the CDC for more than a year (and was fully aware of the chaotic nature of the program) replaced Jack Adler as director a few months later, in 1992. He had previously written to the director outlining his concerns. Frieden had leadership skills, was unafraid of confrontation, relished a major problem, and had an insider's knowledge of the deep problems within the bureau. He had completed his public health thesis on New York City's tuberculosis control in the mid-1980s while at Columbia University and had spent his internship at Columbia Presbyterian, where he had been exposed to increasing numbers of tuberculosis cases. While an EIS officer he had investigated several nosocomial outbreaks of tuberculosis. In addition to being acutely aware of the importance of such outbreaks in the epidemic, he was also, along with others including Karen Brudney and Wafaa El-Sadr in Harlem, fully aware of the more sinister problem that was less amenable to a "quick fix": The increasing burden of multidrug-resistant tuberculosis.

Both Frieden and Fujiwara were funded and employed by the CDC, and both used this fact to make changes. Due to the bureau's poor reputation, without CDC authority Frieden and Fujiwara would have found it all but impossible to achieve the urgent changes required. In fact, shortly after they started, both identified themselves as CDC employees rather than the city's Bureau of Tuberculosis Control representatives. This, they both felt, gave them much-needed credibility with others in the medical profession so that change could be rapidly effected.

PUBLIC HEALTH RESPONSE AND "DELINQUENT" PATIENTS

Failures in surveillance, spread in congregate settings, and failures of treatment completion were at the heart of the public health problem. In January 1992 the New York Academy of Medicine, with the support of the United Hospital Fund, convened a meeting of experts chaired by David Rothman, professor of History at Columbia University and an acknowledged authority on the historical limits on civil liberties in the public health sphere. The group assessed the need for single-disease institutions and "the difficult question of whether those who do not comply with regimens should be confined."[28] They concluded that involuntary commitment to one or two disease-specific facilities was an appropriate policy. This conclusion was based on a number of considerations.

First, "the highly contagious nature of tuberculosis." They and others proposed that "without a special facility for confinement, those at the bottom of the social ladder will be twice penalized, the deprivations of confinement being multiplied by an increased likelihood of exposure to disease" from tuberculosis patients confined while awaiting trial or serving criminal sentences.[29] That is, it was felt that those residing in congregate settings such as prisons and shelters should not have to bear the added burden of potentially being exposed to individuals with tuberculosis who had declined treatment and either relapsed and become infectious or never become uninfectious.

Second, the committee accepted the suggestion by Karen Brudney and Jay Dobkin, clinicians in Harlem, that "Delinquent patients are the core of New York City's TB problem."[30] This suggestion was a preview of later sentiments expressed by the city's public health authorities that "recalcitrant" individuals had to be encouraged to comply with treatment or removed from posing a threat. The chairman of the committee later explained that "Patients [should] be taught and encouraged to follow treatment regimens."[31]

Third, the committee recommended that general hospitals were not appropriate places for patients to be detained, because it would be too costly, disruptive, and was not in keeping with the general ethos of general hospitals.

The committee also suggested that the single-disease facility should be small (as opposed to the public health authority's recommendation, which estimated a need for 200 beds) and that prior to being detained, each patient should be given a trial of directly observed therapy. Committee members recognized that, with this measure, some patients would be lost to follow-up and avoid commitment, but they reasoned that the alternative—immediate incarceration without a trial of DOT—would violate personal liberty and perhaps be unconstitutional because a less restrictive alternative had not been used or attempted. The committee insisted that involuntary commitment be used solely with those who had demonstrated their noncompliance by their actions, not be merely dependent on the supposition of health authority officials. Release from detention should occur, the committee recommended, "when residents no longer pose a threat to the health of others, that is, when they have demonstrated their ability to comply with treatment regimens or when they have been cured of the disease."[32] The committee assumed, therefore, that the association between compliance and public risk was clear. It did not explain how detainees were to demonstrate compliance. A consistent problem faced by those responsible for maintaining the extension of detention has been how autonomous compliance can be predicted on release; almost certainly this has been a contributing factor in maintaining detention of many patients until completion of treatment.

There were two clear practical problems in using a coercive measure such as detention. First, there were no facilities immediately available, and second, the legal framework was thought to be insufficiently robust to withstand a court challenge. Both of these issues were addressed and remedied soon thereafter.

In the spring of 1992, again with the support of the United Hospital Fund, a Working Group was convened by experts in medicine, public health, law, ethics, and public policy to examine the implications of the tuberculosis epidemic from these disciplinary standpoints. They concentrated on addressing problems related to screening for HIV, treatment, and the protection of those in congregate settings, and came up with a series of recommendations that were subsequently published, along with comments from dissenters.[33] In essence, they took a utilitarian stance. They rejected the need for mandatory HIV testing for those with or at risk of tuberculosis and they called on "notions of decency" and "the moral obligation of employers and employees" and the Occupational Safety and Health Act (OSHA) to demand that workplaces be safe from the risk of tuberculosis. The discussion regarding tuberculosis in congregate settings was limited. Recommendations for prisons, shelters, and hospitals stressed the importance of *employee* protection rather than prisoner, client, or patient protection. The group reiterated the guiding principle that the state has an obligation "to protect the health of the public" and that there was a legal basis "for restricting the liberty of those with TB and other infectious diseases that seriously threaten the public health." They agreed with Rothman's committee that detention "beyond infectiousness until cure" was an appropriate response to those failing to comply with treatment and highlighted the need for the provision of adequate and available treatment for allied medical problems that might be expected to inhibit antituberculosis treatment compliance. As part of the program to enhance compliance they advocated universal DOT, such that all patients with tuberculosis should be enrolled in the program. Mark Barnes, associate commissioner, dissented from this view in part because he felt those who were not homeless and who did not have health insurance "would be unnecessarily burdened by this requirement [having] to spend hours waiting for directly observed therapy in over-extended public facilities."[34] Ultimately, as shall be seen, Barnes's view that DOT should be limited prevailed.

The group stressed the need for adequate housing, social services, and psychiatric treatment for patients in order to enhance compliance. Finally, in its conclusion the group remarked that underlying the tuberculosis problem the "social conditions of poverty and overcrowding that give rise to TB today are not so very different from those in the nineteenth and early twentieth centuries" and "overcrowded shelters, prisons, and jails stand as acute reminders of social failure. These conditions are not foreordained; they are predictable consequences of social and political neglect. The resurgence of TB is but one symptom of the failure to provide humane and adequate living conditions for all Americans."[35]

In its effort to stem the epidemic, the city's public health institutions focused on the development of a framework from which a number of agencies within the city could coordinate the response, producing ultimately what was hoped would be a comprehensive plan for tuberculosis control. A "TB Blueprint" outlining the framework and objectives was drawn up. In October 1992 approximately 400 city employees met for three days to clarify the approach that was to be used. The participants came from a number of mayoral offices, including the Department of Health (DOH), the Health and Hospitals Corporation (HHC), the Department of Correction (DOC), the Human Resources Administration (HRA), the Office of Management and Budget (OMB), and the Office of Operations. One of the most important issues, addressed early, included overcoming bureaucratic inertia and enabling those who needed resources, both equipment and staff, to get them quickly, without having to go through the normally slow process previously required by the city. Hiring new health department employees was a priority. The bureau had $10 million, which was going to be lost (returned to the CDC) if it was not spent, 200 vacancies, and not a single named candidate. "It turned out that just about everything that could be going wrong with the hiring process was going wrong, including much of it within the Health Department."[36] As Frieden noted at the time, if the bureaucratic hurdles couldn't be surmounted, "all else will fail completely."[37]

It is clear that there were a number of areas of concern to the public health officials. Many of these, such as poverty, overcrowding, the criminal justice system, and broad economic inequities, they had frustratingly little influence over. Public health officials, therefore, not surprisingly, principally addressed four narrowly focused areas: (1) improvements in infection control in congregate settings to reduce nosocomial spread; (2) reducing new cases by screening and offering preventive treatment to those at risk of relapse; (3) improving completion-of-treatment rates of those with active disease; and (4) management of persistently noncompliant patients.[38]

Substantial extra funding was gained from city, state, and federal sources. New York City increased its total funding for tuberculosis care from $4 million in 1988 to more than $40 million by 1994. In addition, capital expenditure of more than $60 million extra in city funding went toward new facilities at Rikers Island. Federal government, through the CDC, supported in particular the expansion of the DOT program. Bureaucratic hurdles for hiring new staff were removed with the mayor's office giving post-audit approval. The staffing of the bureau increased from just over 50 in 1979, to 144 in 1988, and to more than 600 in 1994, most of these DOT outreach workers who "traveled to patients' homes and workplaces, as well as to street corners, bridges, subway stations, park benches, and even 'crack dens' in abandoned buildings, to ensure that patients were appropriately treated."[39] The number of staff working in Department of Health Tuberculosis Clinics increased from 59 in 1985 to 266 in 1996 (see figure 4.2), and whereas these clinics provided services for only about 5 percent of the yearly reported cases in 1992, after changes were initiated the clinics began to provide care for about one-third of the city's cases.[40] Overall the cost of the epidemic and the response was put at more than $1 billion in 1995, just three years after the control program was reinvigorated.[41]

INFECTION CONTROL IN CONGREGATE SETTINGS

Following several outbreaks in hospitals in New York and elsewhere, infection control in hospitals improved with the recognition of the potential threat to both patients and staff. In 1993, $8.5 million was allocated to 11 hospitals for construction of isolation facilities. This resulted in nearly 400 isolation beds in the city.[42] Hospitals rapidly introduced ventilation systems to minimize the spread of bacteria, ultraviolet irradiation and air filtration to decontaminate air, and

FIGURE 4.2

Growth in New York City Department of Health tuberculosis clinic staff

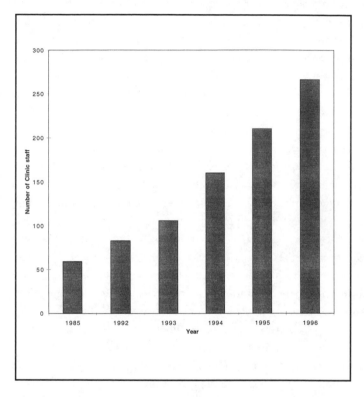

Source: Bureau of Tuberculosis Control, New York City Department of Health.

improved the use of specialized masks to both limit the production of infectious aerosols from patients and to prevent inhalation by others.[43] These efforts appear to have been successful. In one example, nosocomial spread of tuberculosis in a teaching hospital all but ceased after recommended control measures were instituted, and there has been little documented in-hospital spread (other than a nursery outbreak) in New York since the guidelines were issued and acted on.[44]

Spread within shelters for the homeless decreased as a result of other measures being implemented around the same time. Many patients using the huge overcrowded shelters, some of which housed 1,000 individuals in close proximity in a single cavernous room, were offered more humane housing if they fulfilled appropriate criteria, that is, they had AIDS. Some individuals with tuberculosis who were not coinfected with HIV were offered alternative accommodation, at least for the duration of their tuberculosis treatment. Others were moved to shelters in which they shared a room with two or three others, such as the Bellevue Shelter, adjacent to Bellevue Hospital, rather than with hundreds (or thousands) of other homeless people. The conditions at the Bellevue Shelter, which offered beds for up to 85 men with tuberculosis who were noninfectious, were improved in 1992, and a shelter for women and their children, Brooklyn Women's Shelter, opened in 1993 with a capacity for 30 residents. Tuberculosis among those using shelters fell dramatically, from 748 cases in 1991 to 293 cases in 1994.[45]

Heightened public anxiety was reflected in the response to tuberculosis spread within the prison system. Mayor Dinkins, his eye on reelection perhaps, earmarked $100 million of city money for the problem, principally on the new Rikers Island facilities, which, it was proposed, would have 140 state-of-the-art isolation units. On January 24, 1992, Dinkins had been ordered by U.S. District Judge Morris Lasker to construct an isolation unit at Rikers Island by May 1 that year, following several deaths within the prison system in 1991 from nosocomially acquired tuberculosis. In 1988 Lasker had ordered that prisoners with tuberculosis be isolated from other inmates but little had been done.[46] From 1990 the Department of Correction spent more than two years attempting to install ultraviolet lighting and negative-pressure ventilation systems in two infirmaries without achieving satisfactory results. Following the death of a prison guard and several inmates from a prison MDRTB outbreak, however, building work on the isolation ward on Rikers Island was commenced at a cost of $450,000 per room.[47] The first 42 units were completed in May 1992, a further 42 units completed in December, and the last 56 beds completed in mid-1993.[48]

Overall, nosocomial spread in hospitals, shelters, and the prison system (which had accounted for more than a third of all MDRTB cases) declined, and this response arguably had the most substantial impact in "turning the tide" of the epidemic.[49]

IMPROVED SCREENING AND PREVENTIVE TREATMENT

Surveillance was enhanced and a central registry ensured that all data reported to the bureau were computerized. More detailed clinical and demographic data were documented more rapidly, and ongoing analysis was instituted internally to detect trends, outbreaks, and laboratory errors earlier. Screening was directed toward those most at risk, particularly HIV positive patients, contacts of those with active disease, immigrants, and drug users. Screening in correctional institutions was improved, as were links with hospitals. Numerous hospital "grand rounds" were presented by senior public health physicians to increase hospital doctors' awareness and knowledge and improve relationships between clinicians and public health physicians. Links with HIV care providers were improved on, as were those providing care to drug users. New mobile and in-clinic X-ray facilities for screening were bought or updated. Preventive treatment programs were advertised in numerous ways. Because of concerns over the efficacy of preventive treatment of multidrug-resistant tuberculosis, city-specific guidelines were formulated and disseminated. Because of confusion over interpretation of and response to tuberculin, particularly in children, guidelines on this too were updated. (Tuberculin is a preparation derived from *M. tuberculosis* that when injected may indicate previous exposure to tubercle bacilli.) Clinician-laboratory communication was enhanced to improve turnaround times for diagnostic confirmation and isolate sensitivity results.

Mandatory screening for high-risk individuals in prisons and homeless shelters was considered but then rejected. Frieden's scribbled response in the margins beside written proposals was that, applied to residents of shelters, this move was "entirely inappropriate."[50] He does not comment on screening of prisoners, but by December 1991 the New York State Department of Correctional Services had already mandated tuberculin testing for all staff and inmates.[51]

IMPROVED COMPLETION OF TREATMENT RATES

Directly observed therapy was the lynchpin of the expanded public health program in response to the epidemic. The Bureau of Tuberculosis Control had set the goal that, by the end of 1992, 500 patients should have begun DOT. In order to achieve this goal, an incentive program had been initiated offering free lunches, travel token reimbursement, and food vouchers. In the 1980s completion-of-treatment rates in New York were in the order of 50 to 60 percent.[52] By November 1992, 476 patients were on DOT, and by the end of December 1992, the goal had been reached.[53] Partly in response to the efforts taking place in New York, in 1993 the Advisory Council for the Elimination of Tuberculosis (ACET) recommended that DOT be considered in all patients receiving treatment from locales that were not achieving 90 percent completion rates of treatment.[54] This recommendation was largely "in response to the dismal record of assuring that those with tuberculosis complete their treatment, the problems of tuberculosis in persons with HIV infection, and the public alarm that attended the emergence of multidrug-resistant tuberculosis in New York."[55] In prisons directly observed therapy was introduced for all inmates. Paula Fujiwara, current director of the Bureau of Tuberculosis Control, has said that the introduction of DOT required "a 'sea-change,' in attitudes of staff in the Bureau, the medical establishment, public health administrators, and patients. There was skepticism and debate on whether DOT should and, perhaps more importantly, could be effective."[56] DOT ultimately became "the standard of care." Physicians in the bureau were required to document if they did *not* place a patient on DOT and "the compelling reason they had not done so; all patients were advised that this method was the best one to cure them and combat the epidemic of tuberculosis."[57]

DOT services were provided by both the city's Department of Health and non-DOH community providers. Non-DOH programs were funded, in part, by New York State Department of Health start-up grants and were sustained by reimbursement through Medicaid. (Some programs also received Ryan White funds, which were channeled through HIV care services.) Unlike preceding years, substantial efforts were made to seek noncompliant individuals and it was through the bureau's "Return to Service Unit" that noncompliant patients would be sought and treatment orchestrated.

NONCOMPLIANT PATIENTS

Experts in working groups and committees as well as city authorities were in agreement that detention facilities for noninfectious, persistently noncompliant patients should be made available. Most had some reservations, but their belief that such facilities would be used and that the measures were necessary is clear. From a philosophical and legal perspective, the expert groups had argued their case convincingly. Frieden, the driving force behind the city's public health response, believed in the necessity of detention. It enhanced public health officials' credibility with both patients and physicians at a time when this, particularly in the case of the medical profession, was crucial.

But Frieden's reservations were illustrated by his comments to the *New York Times* at the height of the epidemic in October 1992: "There have been calls to quarantine patients or lock them up. I know there will be more because when people are scared they grab for a simple answer, and locking sick people away is a simple answer. Simple, quick and wrong."[58] Moreover, handwritten scribbles in drafts of "Blueprint" documents also point to his concerns, that detention might be used too hastily and for the wrong reasons.[59] A further example, provided years later, of his commitment and sensitivity to social justice concerns was explained to me by lawyer Rose Gasner, head of regulatory affairs at the bureau. She was principle author of a paper describing the city's experience with legal sanctions that was provisionally entitled "NYC's Experience Using Legal Action Against Nonadherent Tuberculosis Patients: 1993–1995." Frieden, who was last (and senior) author, had commented: "Rose, we're not against patients, we're against the bacillus!" The title of the paper was changed to reflect this idea.[60] In 1993 Frieden's concerns regarding civil liberty and social justice issues were ultimately, however, assuaged by his sense of urgency, the magnitude of the problem, and his belief that detention of some was a necessary measure to protect the public health from the spread of disease.

By September 1993 the problem of lack of facilities and the legal constraints involved in incarcerating those who were noninfectious had been remedied. Twenty-five beds, under city control, at Coler/Goldwater Memorial Hospital on Roosevelt Island, were designated for noninfectious tuberculosis patients. Shortly after they opened in September, the number of designated beds increased to 29 with an additional 14 beds available (43 in total) should the need arise.[61] Bellevue Hospital, a city public hospital, opened a 21-bed unit for the detention of infectious patients in addition to updating negative-pressure facilities of its other rooms at around the same time.[62]

CHANGING PUBLIC HEALTH REGULATIONS

Ultimately, many physicians felt the threat of detention was the measure which "encouraged" compliance with DOT, particularly for the more chaotic individuals, and this view was mirrored by the city health officials. Most broadly agreed that "There needs to be a credible threat of detention behind DOT use."[63] Some saw that the role of detention was "to set an example, analogous to IRS picking a small proportion of individuals to audit and making an example of those who defraud."[64] Others were more circumspect: "Detention is analogous to the death penalty as a threat to change behavior. Does the threat of the death penalty deter murderers?"[65] But those holding the latter view were in a minority.

This section describes how the public health regulations were amended, such that detention of noninfectious individuals could be authorized.

Given the perceived changing needs of the public health authorities at that time, the Department of Health and the Board of Health amended the New York City code in April 1993. The purpose of this amendment was to "articulate with greater precision the compulsory measures available to the Department to control the spread of tuberculosis and infection of new cases" and to clarify the commissioner's authority to detain individuals with active tuberculosis who presented a threat to the public health, either because they posed a direct threat of transmission, that is, an immediate threat, or because their noncompliance with treatment might lead to the redevelopment of infectious tuberculosis.[66]

Historically the authority to detain individuals in New York City had been granted by section 11.55 of the New York City Health Code. This authority, although not specifically applying to tuberculosis, gave the commissioner of health broad powers and allowed her, "upon determining that the health of others is endangered," to order the detention of an individual.[67] Another section, 11.47, had been adopted in 1959; although it related specifically to tuberculosis, it provided no authority for detention. This resided within section 11.55. As Mark Barnes, the associate commissioner for policy, and Carlos Ball, counsel for HIV and tuberculosis policy, pointed out, by 1992 the Department of Health was concerned that section 11.55 did "not provide a standard for determining whether detention is appropriate, nor does it provide the detainee with procedural rights."[68] There were concerns that if a constitutional challenge had been brought against section 11.55, it could have been found unconstitutional both because of its vagueness and procedural failings.

What were the arguments advanced for this regulatory change? On October 6, 1992, Frieden made a presentation to the New York City Board of Health outlining the epidemiology of tuberculosis in the city, the new efforts being made to control the epidemic, the implications of noncompliance, and the case for expanding the DOT program. He remarked that noncompliance was the most important problem facing tuberculosis control efforts in New York City and elsewhere, and he highlighted the ideal that all patients should receive directly observed therapy: "we need to reinvigorate our efforts to assure that every patient with active tuberculosis completes treatment."[69] He bemoaned the fact that the detention of patients up until then had been ineffective as a means of disease management and pointed out that only 2 patients out of 33 recently detained had completed treatment and that the then current practice was to detain patients only while they were infectious. With regard to the role of detention, he went on: "for a small number of patients, care in a secure facility may be critical, to protect patients' families and communities, as well as these patients themselves." He noted that "persistently noncompliant patients face a daunting array of problems: homelessness, drug addiction and schizophrenia," and he concluded by highlighting the problems noncompliant patients may face. But he also stressed patients' personal responsibilities and social injustices. He suggested that "while these patients must accept responsibility for their actions, society must also accept responsibility for creating and allowing to flourish the conditions which promote noncompliance: poverty, homelessness, drug abuse, lack of access to medical care, and mental illness." He then continued:

> Although society is, in part, responsible for the situation, this doesn't mean no action should be taken. To continue to allow these individuals to infect others compounds social injustice with deplorable inaction. As individuals, these patients must accept responsibility for completing treatment of tuberculosis. As public health leaders, we must work to establish a context within which such treatment can

occur. As a society, we must assure that these patients complete their treatment and that the social dislocations which have led to their current situation are reversed.

He concluded by calling for the detention of noncompliant individuals both to protect the public and because of the deterrent effect it would have on other patients who might "contemplate" not complying with treatment.[70]

On the same day as Frieden made his presentation, Kenneth Ong, deputy commissioner for disease intervention, wrote to Margaret Hamburg, commissioner of health, outlining the reasons for amending the regulations. These were:

- To articulate with greater precision the compulsory measures available to the Department to control the spread of tuberculosis and infection of new cases;
- To articulate the standards by which the Department will be guided in exercising compulsory measures;
- To ensure that the framework in which the Department acts is governed and guided by sound principles of procedural due process and respect for civil liberties; and
- To modernize the medical elements and terminology for evaluation of patients for tuberculosis.[71]

The board subsequently, in outlining the current status of the epidemic, commented that it had "documented numerous circumstances of patients with active untreated or incompletely treated pulmonary tuberculosis, living in crowded homes or dwellings where transmission to friends and family members sharing living space has occurred."[72]

The department later clarified the circumstances when detention and isolation for individuals with active *infectious* tuberculosis might be ordered. This included persons living in a setting where transmission was likely to occur and persons with active infectious tuberculosis who refused to submit voluntarily to evaluation and treatment.

The original four subsections of section 11.47, (a) to (d), were left largely unchanged (although reduced to three subsections). A further seven subsections, (d) to (j), were added. Subsection (d) set out the enforceable orders at the disposal of the commissioner with regard to the threat to the public health of a case or suspected cases of tuberculosis. Subsection (d) allowed that "*the Commissioner may issue any orders he or she deems necessary to protect the public health* or the health of any other person, and may make application to a court for enforcement of such orders" (emphasis added). In addition, the provisions of Subsection (d) authorized the commissioner to order:

- Physical examinations of cases having or suspected of having active tuberculosis.
- A person with active tuberculosis to complete a course of treatment and follow necessary contagion precautions.
- A person with active tuberculosis to follow a course of DOT.
- The removal and detention of a person (i) who has active tuberculosis that is infectious; and (ii) "where the Department finds, based on recognized infection control principles, that there is a *substantial likelihood* such person may transmit to others tuberculosis because of his or her inadequate separation from others."
- The removal and detention of a person (i) who has active tuberculosis; and (ii) "*where there is a substantial likelihood, based on such person's past or present behavior, that he or she can not* [sic] *be relied upon to participate in and/or to complete an appropriate prescribed course of medication for tuberculosis* and/or, if necessary, to follow required contagion precautions for tuberculosis. Such behavior may include, but is not limited to, refusal or failure to take medication for tuberculosis, or refusal or failure to keep appointments for treating tuberculosis, or refusal or failure to complete treatment for tuberculosis, or disregard for contagion precautions for tuberculosis." (emphasis added)[73]

Subsections (e) to (j) are described in the appendix.

In essence, therefore, the amended regulations emphasized compliance with treatment (and, largely by assumption, the public health threat) rather than responding to a defined threat to the public posed by noncompliant individuals. Furthermore, with regard to due process, unlike the recommendations of the committee of the New York Academy of Medicine,[74] the regulations did not mandate that less restrictive alternatives be attempted before detaining an individual if the commissioner deemed such measures "necessary to protect the public health."

RESPONSE TO THE PROPOSAL TO AMEND THE REGULATIONS

The New York City Tuberculosis Working Group (principally composed of advocates for people living with HIV infection and AIDS and for people living in poverty) responded to the proposals reiterating their comments made earlier in 1992, by pointing out that, although they agreed that compliance with medical care was a matter of personal responsibility, in the absence of access to adequate housing, primary healthcare, and adequate substance abuse services, it was "inappropriate and premature to discuss the detention" of noninfectious patients.[75] They emphasized the need for systems to improve voluntary treatment compliance. Furthermore, if civil detention was to occur, they demanded that two principles should be complied with.

First, in the case of any individual with tuberculosis, it should be shown by "a factual finding that he or she presents a significant risk of harm to others."[76] This, they said, was commensurate with section 504 of the Rehabilitation Act, Title II of the Americans with Disabilities Act (ADA). They went on further to comment that a *speculative* risk should not justify the imposition of these public health measures and that the risk, based on an individualized judicial inquiry, should be *actual*. Later Mike Isbell, a civil rights advocate who contributed to the working group, also commented that "even if the significant risk standard were not technically applicable to TB detention orders, it is still unclear why the City would refrain from including the standard in the proposed law. After all, why would the City ever want to detain someone who posed no significant risk to the public health."[77] Indeed.

The second principle they argued was that under constitutional due process protections and the ADA, no person should be detained until authorities have made a good faith attempt to employ every available less restrictive means to reduce that person's risk of harm to an insignificant level. This, they suggested, made the city beholden "to develop and properly fund a social service infrastructure" that could appropriately meet the needs of those with tuberculosis.[78] They also reiterated the suggestion that any decisions should be individualized and not dependent on broad categorical characteristics, such as homelessness, alcoholism, or drug dependency.

In conclusion, perhaps anticipating David Rothman's later comment that detention facilities for patients with tuberculosis "stand as a monument to the inadequacy of more imaginative and benevolent public programs," the group reflected that, by scapegoating vulnerable noncompliant patients, public health policymakers were perpetuating "the neglect and denial that have produced the resurgence in TB."[79]

PUBLIC HEARING

At the public hearing that followed in December 1992 to discuss the proposed amendments, the vast majority of those who spoke, including nearly all the physicians involved, supported the proposed regulatory amendments. This was not surprising—many had received reminders of the meeting from those eager to see the proposed amendments supported publicly. Most, like Jay Dobkin, emphasized individual responsibilities: "These changes [to the regulations] send a strong signal to patients, doctors and society at large that no one has the right to recklessly endanger the health of others, especially when simple means are available to control and cure the disease."[80] Others, such as Donald Armstrong of Sloan Kettering Medical Center, mirrored Lee Reichman's comments earlier in the year regarding staffing of hospitals when he stressed the dangers healthcare workers faced from working in New York. He feared workers would leave the city "because they're afraid of TB and afraid that we are not taking action in order to protect them from tuberculosis."[81]

Some, including perhaps the more liberal-minded participants, highlighted the need for adequate legal protections and reiterated the comments made by the New York Academy of Medicine Committee that less restrictive alternatives should be exhausted before detention was used. A few of the civil rights advocates, including representatives of the Commission on Human Rights, Lambda Legal Defense Fund (an organization concerned with gay rights), and the Association of the Bar of the City of New York, called for the department to prove, in each case, that the individual to be detained posed a substantial risk to others.

Most of those who spoke at the hearing, however, accepted that those who failed to comply with treatment automatically posed a substantial public health threat. The city had involved the New York Civil Liberties Union (NYCLU) at an early stage in drafting the amendments. This was astute in so much as it reduced the possibility that perhaps the most powerful civil rights group would mount an early constitutional challenge to the amendments. Although the NYCLU opposed the proposed amendments, it emphasized perceived failures in due process rather than weaknesses in the determination of public health threat.[82]

Ethicists Nancy Dubler and Ron Bayer both commented on the proposals. As he had when he had been a member of the United Hospital Fund's Working Group, Bayer argued a utilitarian position, noting that "No conception of the ethics of public health would provide ground for objecting to such measures, since no conception of ethics would find objectionable restrictions on individuals who could pose a threat to the health and safety of others. Indeed, on some readings of the ethics of public health, it would represent a moral failure and a dereliction of professional responsibility not to act when individuals pose a threat to others." But he also went on: "In recognizing that the control of tuberculosis requires extension of the responsibility of the DOH to the noninfectious state of active disease, there is an implicit recognition of the responsibility to provide the conditions that will enhance patient cooperation," although he recognized this task was "beyond the purview of the Department of Health." Nancy Dubler noted that although "tuberculosis is a threat to the health of individuals and to the well-being of the public . . . in a larger sense, it is a challenge to our notion of community, to the fairness we will demand and the repression we will tolerate in pursuit of the health of the public." She too highlighted the obligations that the introduction of the amendments put on the other agencies of government for patients with tuberculosis.[83]

DEPARTMENT OF HEALTH RESPONSE

The Department of Health responded to these comments. On the issue that all available less restrictive means should be exhausted, it agreed to perform an "individualized assessment and give priority to less restrictive treatment alternatives where appropriate (that is, where there is a substantial probability of success) and available." Despite the earlier report from the New York Academy of Medicine and the criticisms arising from the public meeting, the department would not, however, set predetermined measures such as compulsory DOT before imposing detention. Instead, it commented that "the Department cannot and should not be required to exhaust a pre-set, rigid hierarchy of alternative measures that would ostensibly encourage voluntary compliance, but then be compelled to wait for the patient to fail each of them," and "interventions must be tailored to the patient's individual circumstances and based on reasonable judgment as to what interventions will best assure treatment until cured." State discretion was required, the department argued, and this was the position it maintained.

Responding to the "significant risk" standard, as defined by the ADA, the department argued that the ADA was "inapplicable to the exercise of public health communicable disease control measures and the exercise of police power." It suggested that the ADA focused on individuals and the immediate risk any individual poses to others, and it did not, in addition, allow an assessment of *aggregate* risk. The inclusion of an assessment of aggregate risk was important because, it said, "emphasis must be placed on the cumulative or likely risk to the public health created by noncompliance with tuberculosis treatment in a number of persons or by a single individual over time." The department recognized that a noncompliant patient may pose only a "small risk directly to the public" but argued, not surprisingly, that the risk increases if many patients fail to comply with treatment. It further acknowledged that noncompliant patients who were noninfectious did not pose an "immediate or imminent threat at a particular point in time" but argued that "over time, it is likely that they will pose a very serious threat to large segments of the public." In support of its argument that aggregate risk should be taken into account, the Department of Health produced the example of a vaccination program for a bacterial or viral disease and the reasoning behind why such programs are compulsory. (Vaccination, as noted in chapter 2, is compulsory in most states of the United States as a condition of admission to school, and parents may constitutionally be convicted of violating the compulsory school attendance law when they attempt to exempt their child; schools cannot legally admit a child without him or her having had the necessary vaccinations or immunizations.) When vaccination levels in the general population fall, although the risk to any one individual is small, the risk to the population as a whole increases substantially. That is, there is "herd protection" when vaccination programs cover a certain proportion of children. The department described as analogous the position of a person with active, noninfectious tuberculosis. It suggested that "if enough cases of partially or incompletely treated cases of tuberculosis occur, we likely will see an increase in prevalence of multidrug-resistant tuberculosis, first in noncompliant patients and then in patients who acquire multidrug-resistant tuberculosis as a primary infection."

In essence, therefore, the Department of Health recognized the assertion that those who are noncompliant with treatment and noninfectious do not pose an immediate threat to public health but argued that to preserve "herd protection," the aggregate risks arising from many individuals failing to comply with treatment meant that any individual who could not or would not comply with appropriate treatment should be detained until he or she no longer posed a public health threat, however small that threat was. The department did not respond to the comments regarding the broader societal questions.[84]

The Amendments to section 11.47 of the New York City Health Code were adopted on March 9, 1993, and made effective on April 29. On March 9, the Board of Health of the Department of Health also passed a "Resolution and Finding" that was not open to public scrutiny or comment before being issued. It resolved that "the potential reactivation of tuberculosis and the development and spread of drug-resistant tuberculosis caused by the failure of tuberculosis patients, whether or not infectious, to complete a course of anti-tuberculosis therapy create a *significant* threat to the public health" (emphasis added). The implicit assumption of threat in the statute (regarding noninfectious individuals) was made explicit only in the Resolution and Finding.

FEDERAL RESPONSE

Six months later, in November 1993, the CDC issued recommendations pertaining to the control of tuberculosis laws. With regard to the commitment of patients with tuberculosis, it suggested that all states should adopt step-by-step interventions beginning with DOT, DOT under a court order, and finally detention. Furthermore, it advised that state laws should permit the involuntary isolation and detention of

noninfectious patients who, after being offered less restrictive alternatives, refuse to comply with a treatment regimen or to complete
treatment. At the time the report was drafted, 42 states permitted the
commitment of patients with tuberculosis with considerable variation in
the legal processes, duration of commitment, and specification of the
state of the disease.[85]

ARE THE AMENDED REGULATIONS CONSTITUTIONAL?

The health board, by emphasizing completion of treatment as the
measure that would ultimately, in practice, determine when detention
orders were issued, managed to sidestep the more complex issue of
determining the threat any individual might pose to the public. Indeed,
on the issue of risk the city appeared to contradict itself. In response to
the comments made at the public hearing, the city acknowledged that
the risk posed at any one time by a noncompliant noninfectious
individual was small. Yet at the time the resolution was adopted, under
the Resolution and Finding published with the notice of adoption (*after*
the public hearing), it was suggested that noncompliance created "the
likelihood of relapse into infectiousness," and the Board of Health
resolved that "the failure of tuberculosis patients . . . to complete a course
of anti-tuberculosis therapy create a *significant* threat to the public
health" (emphasis added). This avoidance of a detailed analysis of the
risks posed by noninfectious individuals was understandable. Much of
what was known (and indeed is known) about the risks of relapse and
infectiousness was simply conjecture, and whereas a court would find it
easier to predict future noncompliance on the basis of past behavior,
experts, and hence the courts, would have difficulty defining the threat
any single individual posed. Moreover, as an individual was detained for
longer periods and complied with treatment for longer, so his or her risk
of relapse would fall and his or her threat to the public health decline.
The courts would therefore have to consider release more favorably as
time went on. But with the emphasis on treatment compliance the
standard would be dependent on behavior, not threat, and release would
be more dependent on the perception and comments of the hospital
health professionals regarding future behavior.

Despite this uncertainty, at some of the court hearings where
background information has been presented regarding the probability of

patients becoming infectious should they fail to comply with treatment, city representatives commented that "If a patient stops taking the appropriate medication before the expiration of these six to nine months . . . the patient will *likely* become infectious again" (emphasis added)[86]; indeed, when pressed, city representatives have at times given precise figures regarding the risk of relapse.[87]

Much of the health department's argument regarding the public health threat hinged on its analogy with vaccination programs. This analogy is erroneous, however. The benefits of vaccination programs rest on active intervention in the mass of individuals to protect the few rather than intervention in the few to protect the mass. Furthermore, in vaccination programs a threshold can be reached whereby, despite less than 100 percent coverage, herd protection is produced. The same cannot be said for a few poorly compliant tuberculosis patients.

So, briefly, what is the legal framework whereby detention of noninfectious persons is justified? The Supreme Court has set constitutional standards that must be met before any individual can be detained.

Statutory Rights of an Individual

Particularized Assessment

As noted in chapter two the Supreme Court has found that, in the case of mental illness, there is "no constitutional basis for confining such persons involuntarily if they are dangerous to no one and can live safely in freedom."[88] The law does not allow an individual to be detained simply because he or she has tuberculosis. Although determining whether an individual with tuberculosis will comply with treatment may be difficult, it is probably easier than predicting future behavior of mentally ill persons or future infectiousness. But depriving a person of their liberty on the basis of a judgment or perception of future noncompliance (as became possible in New York City) rather than on the person's own record of compliance with treatment may be a violation of fundamental notions of due process. Furthermore, the prediction of an individual's future behavior with regard to compliance must not constitutionally be based on his or her status (e.g., HIV status, employment status, whether he or she is an alcoholic or crack addict). As well as being unconstitutional, such classifications also serve poorly as indicators of future adherence to treatment.[89] Yet in making judgments about future behavior, officials often have little else upon which to base their judgments. Basing detention on an assessment of compliance rather than an assessment of threat is, therefore, probably unconstitutional.

Less restrictive alternatives

The Board resisted the use of specific "hurdles" before which an individual must stumble before being detained, even though the New York Academy of Medicine, advocates' groups, and subsequently the CDC all asserted that certain defined measures, such as compulsory DOT orders, should be used before detention orders are issued so that failure to comply with less restrictive alternatives can be formally documented. The board's argument was based on a concern that some individuals, who *could be predicted* to fail, would do so and not comply even when offered less restrictive alternatives to detention. Yet most would agree that predicting compliance is an uncertain science. And therefore, by extension, predicting those who will fail to comply when offered support is also a difficult and uncertain business. Does this approach meet with the doctrine of offering "less restrictive alternatives"? The measures "deemed necessary" by the health commissioner, if they mean detention before other less restrictive alternatives have been offered, may therefore also be unconstitutional. Several individuals have been detained before less restrictive alternatives have been offered them.

Procedural Rights

The amendments that were adopted clarified the position of the board and the individual with regard to the authority held by the commissioner. What is not clear, however, is whether the "layers of professional review" and the "concerns of family and friends" that should provide adequate protection for those civilly detained do so.[90] The protection offered the individual may be inadequate because the courts may fail to critically analyze scientific opinion and the patient's family and friends may fail to offer support and protection. Most patients detained are socially isolated, and since 1993 only one of more than two hundred noninfectious patients detained by the city has been released through a court hearing.

Americans with Disabilities Act (ADA)

Some legal scholars have suggested that the traditional exercise of public health powers has, because its approach treats unequally those with communicable diseases, been discriminatory and favored the public interest rather than individual civil rights. They and others have advanced the notion that the antidiscrimination mandate of the ADA, which requires *reasonable accommodations* as a component of equitable treatment for persons with disabilities, is the standard under which the public interest and individual civil rights should be assessed.[91]

The ADA was intended to provide "a clear and comprehensive national mandate for the elimination of discrimination against individuals with disabilities."[92] It targets discrimination in employment (Title 1), public services (Title II), public accommodations and services operated by private entities (Title III), and telecommunications (Title IV). But does it offer safeguards for individuals with tuberculosis threatened with detention, and likewise does it protect the public health?

In arguing that the ADA should be the statute under which those who are detained should be examined, advocates have argued that the ADA not only prohibits discrimination against persons with disease in employment and public accommodations, but Title II means that the ADA applies to all public services. These services include all actions by state and local governments, including those of public health departments. The argument hinges on two points.

The first point is, that individuals with tuberculosis are "qualified" for protection under the ADA. It has been argued that such individuals are qualified to receive the protection afforded by the ADA.[93] In the context of the ADA, the term "qualified," although not defined in Title II, means that the individual must meet all of the performance or eligibility criteria for the particular position, service, or benefit and that "reasonable accommodations" must be met to enable that person to meet the performance or eligibility criteria. Although Titles I and IV are not directly applicable to public services, legal scholars have suggested that Congress did not intend to force public institutions to accept individuals who "pose a direct threat to the health or safety of others."[94] If one accepts this sensible assertion, then the "direct threat" standard is critical in determining whether an individual with tuberculosis is qualified for protection under the ADA once "reasonable accommodations" have eliminated the risk of communicating the disease to others. Ball and Barnes, in opposing the claim of legal scholar Larry Gostin and others that the ADA was the appropriate review vehicle, have argued that detention for the protection of the public health does not involve state entities providing "benefits of services, programs, or activities" as delineated in the act and therefore those with tuberculosis threatened with detention should not be eligible to receive protection under it. In support of this stand, they further argued that it was not the intention of Congress, when the act was drafted, "to interfere with state and local public health measures aimed at curbing transmission of disease."[95]

The second point concerns whether individuals with tuberculosis are disabled. Even if the court agreed that the standard of the ADA was applicable because individuals with tuberculosis are "qualified" for protection, it still would need to recognize tuberculosis, even asymptomatic, partially treated tuberculosis, as a disability. Under the ADA, a disability is defined as "a physical or mental impairment that substantially limits one or more of the major life activities."[96] As of mid-1999 it is unclear whether an individual with asymptomatic tuberculosis is disabled under this definition.

Following the legal case of *School Board of Nassau County, Florida v. Arline,* communicable diseases, including tuberculosis, may be considered a disability. In this case the Supreme Court upheld Gene Arline's case that she had been unlawfully dismissed. Ms. Arline was an elementary school teacher who, from 1966 until 1979, had taught in Nassau County, Florida. She had been dismissed after suffering a third relapse of tuberculosis within two years. Those responsible for dismissing her had argued that she posed a threat to her students and, as such, was ineligible for protection from discrimination under the ADA. This case, therefore, assessed discrimination in employment, not detention for noncompliance. Furthermore, although having a disability automatically confers protection under the ADA, simply having tuberculosis does not. As Chief Justice William Rehnquist noted when dissenting from the decision made in *Arline,* the central question in the case was "whether discrimination on the basis of contagiousness constitutes discrimination 'by reason of . . . handicap.'"[97] And the answer from *Arline* was that contagiousness did not confer handicap, although one could be handicapped and have a contagious disease. In a footnote, in *Arline* it was made clear, despite Chief Justice Rehnquist's dissent, that the judgment regarding protection under the ADA for asymptomatic individuals with contagious diseases would be left for another day: "We . . . do not reach, the questions whether a carrier of a contagious disease . . . could be considered to have a physical impairment, or whether such a person could be considered, solely on the basis of contagiousness, a handicapped person as defined by the Act." Ultimately, therefore, it is unclear whether, even if qualified by dint of detention in a public hospital, all those with asymptomatic tuberculosis would be viewed as disabled and therefore be eligible for protection under the ADA.

Some legal scholars had hoped that a Supreme Court ruling in 1998 would clarify of some of these issues. This ruling related to an asymptomatic HIV-infected dental patient, Sidney Abbott, who was denied treatment in a dental office on the basis of her HIV status. The Court ruled that asymptomatic infection (HIV in this case) was a disability because it was judged that HIV infection is an "impairment [which] affects a major life activity," notably reproduction.[98] The decision went on, "In the end, the disability definition does not turn on personal choice. When significant limitations result from the impairment, the definition is met even if the difficulties are not insurmountable." Because the ruling hinged on impairment resulting from the impact of HIV on reproduction, and therein the risk to public health, it sheds little light on how to view recalcitrant individuals with asymptomatic tuberculosis. For the ADA to be operative, the impairment must "affect a major life activity," and it is difficult to see what major life activity asymptomatic tuberculosis impairs (likewise to some extent asymptomatic HIV infection). In the case of Sidney Abbott, Chief Justice Rehnquist and three other Justices dissented, arguing that reproduction was not a major life activity—it is not "essential in the day-to-day existence of a normally functioning individual." And in *Arline,* impairment was deemed to result from a "physiological disorder affecting the respiratory system" that also affected her ability to work (in a school). Thus this ruling does not clarify how asymptomatic noninfectious patients could fall under the purview of the ADA, unless it was through having "a record of such an impairment" or "being regarded as having such an impairment."[99] If, however, it is assumed that even partially treated noninfectious tuberculosis does affect a major life activity, and individuals so affected are "eligible" for protection, they must still not pose a direct threat to others.

What is "direct threat"? Consistent with *Arline,* it is defined as *"a significant risk* to the health or safety of others" that cannot be eliminated by reasonable accommodation (emphasis added).[100] The assessment of risk, under disability law, must rest on carefully reasoned judgments based on well-established scientific information, and not "irrational fears, speculation, stereotypes, or pernicious mythologies."[101] In *Arline,* the Supreme Court set out four factors that should be weighed when judging the threat or risk to others an individual with a communicable disease poses. These include: (1) how the disease is transmitted; (2) how long the carrier is infectious; (3) what the potential harm to others is; and (4) what the probability the disease will be transmitted and will cause harm is.

Furthermore, the risk must be determined on an individual basis, including confirmation that the individual has tuberculosis, that it is *transmissible,* and that there is evidence that the person will engage in "dangerous" behavior. As Gostin has noted, there is no reason why the application of the ADA is limited to present infectiousness, but "direct" risks should include risks that are reasonably foreseeable.[102] So, in the case of a noninfectious individual, the "carrier" is, by definition, not infectious. And the potential harm and the possibility of that harm occurring are uncertain, but probably small, and diminishing as treatment continues. The ADA makes plain that a "clear, defined standard, which requires actual proof of significant risk to others" is required; in the case of noninfectious tuberculosis, the risk may not be obvious.

It is therefore unclear whether the amended regulations would withstand rigorous constitutional examination. The regulations fail to demand a less restrictive alternative to detention before it is instituted and give the commissioner of health considerable discretionary powers. Detention may be sanctioned simply on the basis of the judgment of future poor compliance with no documented evidence of poor compliance in the past required. When weighing the merits of the different arguments for and against protection by the ADA for those detained, it is worth remembering (as Barnes and Ball did for the city) the sobering words of Chief Justice Rehnquist in *Arline:* "Congress has legislated directly in the area of contagious diseases. . . . Congress has also . . . left significant leeway to the States, which have enacted a myriad of public health statutes designed to protect against the introduction and spread of contagious diseases." Although it is unclear whether review under the

ADA of a case would be upheld, history suggests that the courts would probably favor the judgment of local public health officials.

CONCLUSION

The seeds of the New York City tuberculosis epidemic of the early 1990s had been sown years before, and their germination had been encouraged by political, public health, and medical neglect. With rates rising dramatically among society's most marginalized, and with outbreaks occurring in prisons, shelters, and hospitals, the public was made aware of the situation in about 1992, as the epidemic reached its peak. The media described the scandal of poor investment in the public health infrastructure and followed the authorities' lead that noncompliant patients posed the greatest threat to the wider community. One key response was to focus on increasing completion-of-treatment rates, and this in turn directed attention to some of the city's most chaotic patients, those unwilling or unable to comply with treatment.

The questions raised included: How could these patients be "encouraged" to complete their treatment? How could they be prevented from posing a public health threat in the face of uncertainty over the magnitude of this threat? And could they be used as an example to persuade others to comply with their treatment? In response, the city chose to regulate for compliance with treatment rather than assess public health threat; in the words of city officials, "the use of detention as a public health intervention [would] not center on the fact that an individual has tuberculosis, but instead, on the fact that she has failed to complete treatment."[103] This approach received wide support both locally and farther afield, including the American academic press. Somewhat surprisingly, academic commentators agreed that the risk to the public should be understood simply as risk based on past behavior of noncompliance rather than estimates of future contagiousness.[104] In pursuing this line of argument, city officials argued that the ADA was an inappropriate statute under which to examine such cases, as it would entail an assessment of public health threat, or "direct threat." But as Gostin pointed out "the argument is circular because the very question the ADA asks is whether the person poses a significant risk to others because of a failure to complete treatment. If the health department can demonstrate a significant risk, it can surely act because the standards of the Act are met."[105] This is similar to the rhetorical point raised by Isbell at the public hearing questioning: Why would "the City ever want to detain someone who posed no significant risk to the public health"?[106]

Irrespective of the details of the arguments for and against using the ADA standard to judge detention, clearly the detention of noncompliant, noninfectious individuals was intended to protect the public health. The problem for those urging detention has been that although noncompliant, noninfectious individuals pose a potentially serious threat—multidrug-resistant tuberculosis—it is neither immediate, quantifiable, or probably substantial. Furthermore, the threat declines the longer any individual is on treatment, and at some point a threshold would be crossed where, if detention were based on the chance of becoming a threat to public health, that patient should be released before treatment is completed even if future compliance is expected to be poor. As a consequence, and in order to maintain the credibility of the *threat* of detention, some individuals have been detained for prolonged periods even though, in all probability, they no longer pose a current or future public health threat. Although the law does not allow for "examples" to be made of some individuals, the regulatory emphasis on compliance rather than threat has allowed this to occur. And this has been the significant change in the public health legal framework. In the case of mental illness and contagious diseases, when an individual threatens the public health, isolation by commitment, detention, or quarantine from the public environs is based on the notion of threat posed rather than failure to comply with treatment. With tuberculosis this ceased to be the case in New York City in 1993. Perhaps not too surprisingly, when one considers the great success of the public health program, the use of coercive measures in support of the response has attracted little attention, and apparently it has been assumed that, because tuberculosis rates have fallen so fast, detention of noncompliant, noninfectious patients was, and is, an appropriate response to recalcitrant patients.

In addition to the uncertainties surrounding the prediction of behavior, there is a moral and legal dilemma, which Thomas Babington Macauley recognized when he wrote the lines quoted at the beginning of this chapter. When an option is not made available, it is impossible for individuals to fail to comply with that option. They must be allowed to fail before being condemned for that failure. This notion applies to both those detained before they have had the chance to fail to comply with treatment, and those individuals detained who are automatically placed on a DOT regime; they can hardly display their willingness to comply and retain their autonomy under such circumstances.

Canute's Apotheosis

But owing to the great spread of this disease, all steps which are taken against the same will have to reckon with the social condition, and, therefore, it must be carefully considered in what way and how far one may go on this road without prejudicing the advantages gained, by unavoidable disturbances and other disadvantages

—Robert Koch, "Die Aetiologie der Tuberkulose," 1882

In 1995 *The New England Journal of Medicine* published a paper by Thomas Frieden and his colleagues entitled "Tuberculosis in New York City—Turning the Tide."[1] The article highlighted the remarkable successes achieved by New York City's Bureau of Tuberculosis Control since the "Blueprint" was enacted under his leadership and documented the 21 percent decline (which had followed more than a decade of year-to-year increases) in the number of cases between 1992 and 1994. The paper emphasized that this decline correlated with the expansion of the directly observed therapy program. Other factors including improvements in infection control, both in hospitals and other congregate settings (not least for the homeless), and the use of detention as a deterrent to encourage compliance were noted to be important influences in the decline. Since 1994 the tide has remained out. Tuberculosis rates have continued to decline (to the astonishment of some international experts), and drug-resistant and multidrug-resistant strains have ceased to be the major cause for concern they were. Furthermore, with

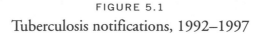

FIGURE 5.1

Tuberculosis notifications, 1992–1997

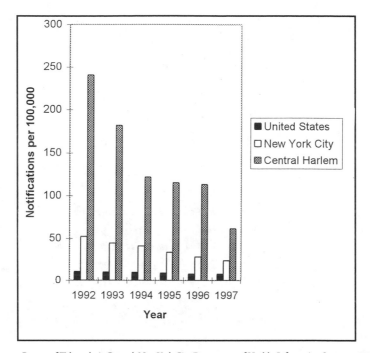

Source: Bureau of Tuberculosis Control, New York City Department of Health; Information Summary 1997.

the national expansion of public health efforts and improved funding for tuberculosis control programs, this decline in tuberculosis rates has been documented across the country. The New York City public health response has been remarkably successful. (See figure 5.1.) The bureau has achieved what Canute could not; it has held back the tide. Chaos has been controlled. But control has required coercion.

SUCCESS

By 1997 the number of tuberculosis cases had fallen to 1,730 per year, 55 percent fewer cases than in 1992. Other evidence confirmed that the control measures were working. Cases of tuberculosis in young children declined (see figure 5.2), and rates of drug resistance and multidrug resistance fell. (See figure 5.3.)[2]

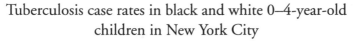

FIGURE 5.2

Tuberculosis case rates in black and white 0–4-year-old
children in New York City

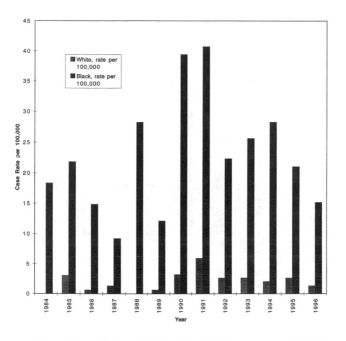

Source: Bureau of Tuberculosis Control, New York City Department of Health.

In deprived poverty-stricken areas, although rates remained above the city average, they also had declined. In 1997 Central Harlem, for example, had 69 cases of tuberculosis (an age-adjusted rate of 61.6 per 100,000) compared to 256 cases in 1992 (an age-adjusted rate of 240.2 per 100,000).[3] The horrendous 1991 tuberculosis incidence rates among blacks (which can be interpreted, with some provisos, as a proxy for rates associated with poverty) declined. Tuberculosis rates in black males in the 35- to 44-year age group were still high in 1997, at 107.2 per 100,000, but were a substantial improvement on the 469.7 per 100,000 rate of 1991.[4] By 1997 the only blip on the control program's "scanner" was tuberculosis in foreign-born individuals. The number of such cases had risen from 872 in 1992 to 1,010 in 1995, a disproportionate rise given falling rates among U.S.-born patients.[5] This occur-

FIGURE 5.3

Cases of multidrug-resistant tuberculosis in New York City

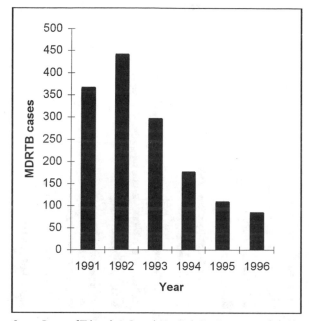

Source: Bureau of Tuberculosis Control, New York City Department of Health.

rence could have been predicted if inadequate port surveillance and poor services for immigrants persisted in concert with the global resurgence of tuberculosis.[6] These trends again reflected national trends.[7] Over the past few years, however, with improved surveillance and targeting of services toward immigrants in the city, cases in foreign-born patients have also declined in number. In 1997, 884 cases were documented.[8]

In prisons the decline in rates was perhaps most dramatic. From 1991 to 1997 there was a greater than 70 percent drop in the number of tuberculosis cases, from 225 per 100,000 to 61 per 100,000, and there have been no new outbreaks since 1993.[9]

Completion-of-treatment rates, not surprisingly, improved from the dismal levels of the late 1980s, where only approximately 50 to 60 percent of patients were completing a course of antituberculosis therapy.[10] Of patients diagnosed in 1996, for example, 93.2 percent completed treatment.[11] Although the number of cases of directly

FIGURE 5.4

Cases of directly observed therapy in New York City

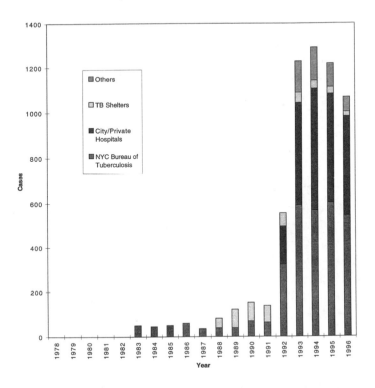

Source: Bureau of Tuberculosis Control, New York City Department of Health.

observed therapy fell since the peak of 1994, the proportion of the total number of cases receiving DOT continued to rise (but has fallen off recently). (See figure 5.4.) Furthermore, DOT has been focused on individuals with multidrug-resistant tuberculosis and pulmonary disease (although the bureau's goal has been to get everyone to take the treatment under observation). In 1997, 77 percent of patients with infectious pulmonary tuberculosis received DOT compared to 72 percent overall, and 87 percent of MDRTB cases received DOT.[12] With this improved control, the prevalence of drug-resistant cases declined, and partly as a consequence, national rates improved.[13] In a report from the Centers for Disease Control and Prevention, the proportion of isolates resistant to isoniazid from patients previously untreated for tuberculosis (i.e., primary resistance) in the city declined from 15 percent in 1993 to 12 percent in 1996. Rates of MDRTB decreased from 9 percent of isolates in 1993 to 5 percent in 1995 and 1996.[14] Other reports from New York City itself also showed a substantial decline in drug-resistant rates.[15]

Despite the expansion of DOT services and the amendments to the public health regulations, many individuals still failed to comply with treatment. Commissioner's orders (i.e., orders issued by the commissioner of health compelling an individual to be examined for suspected tuberculosis, complete treatment, be mandated to be on a DOT program, or be detained) were issued to encourage compliance. (See figure 5.5.) In the first two years after the regulatory amendments, approximately 2 percent of tuberculosis patients were subjected to regulatory intervention, one-quarter of whom had MDRTB. During this period about 1 percent of tuberculosis patients were detained. Compared to mandatory DOT, those detained (both infectious and noninfectious individuals) had been less compliant and had been less willing to accept voluntary DOT. Ninety-six percent of patients issued orders, either for mandatory DOT or detention, completed treatment. For many of those issued mandatory DOT orders who continued to fail to comply, the bureau policy was to issue a letter warning of the consequences. That is, individuals were forewarned that they would be detained if compliance did not improve. This measure, it appears, was successful in improving treatment compliance in most patients.[16]

Between 1993 and 1995, 97 of 116 patients detained long-term were held at Goldwater Memorial Hospital, on the East River's Roosevelt Island. The median duration of stay was 23 weeks, and varied from 2 weeks to 138 weeks. Less than a third of those who were held long-term were released before completing their treatment, and all except one release resulted from a bureau decision to hasten release rather than through a court hearing. Several patients died while detained, most from complications of AIDS. Few succumbed to tuberculosis, which, considering the burden of cases with MDRTB, highlights the excellent clinical care the patients received. Many of those at death's door rallied and left detention healthier than they had been for years. Those detained were demographically similar (other than the frequency of homelessness) to those requiring less draconian coercive measures (i.e., those issued commissioner's orders for DOT). Detainees

FIGURE 5.5

Commissioner's orders for DOT and detention in New York City

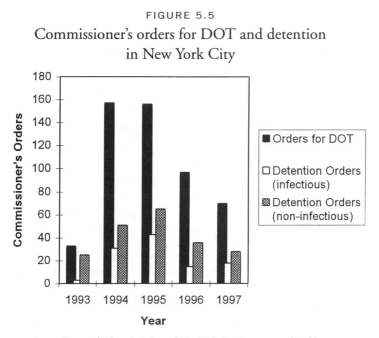

Source: Bureau of Tuberculosis Control, New York City Department of Health.

were overwhelmingly from minority populations (less than 10 percent were white), and nearly 90 percent were born in the United States. More than 60 percent had been homeless, more than half had spent time in prison, and illicit drug use had been a frequent pastime for most. Those detained were more likely than those simply given DOT orders to have respiratory disease and to have been infectious for longer periods.[17] The characteristics of patients being detained has changed over time in a revealing manner. Patients "fail" at compliance "hurdles" fewer times now than they did in the past before they end up in Goldwater Hospital. In 1993, perhaps because of the backlog of chaotic patients, it was not unusual to see patients who had been admitted to a hospital with tuberculosis many times, sometimes more than 10, and then, on discharge, fail to comply with treatment. In 1997 and 1998 most patients failed to comply with treatment only once or twice.[18] The psychological character of the patients has changed too. Many patients in the first couple of years were belligerent, angry, and disruptive. More were alcoholic, many had had convictions for violent offenses, and violence within the unit was not uncommon. More recently patients being detained are more passive and resigned, although illicit drug abuse is still a frequent factor in their lives. Disruption of the unit occurs less often. Whether this reflects the changing nature of the population with tuberculosis, improvements in the ability of the bureau staff to determine those who are likely to persistently fail to comply, or a more streamlined process of detention is not clear but is quite likely a combination of all three possibilities.

Whether some clinicians resort to detention earlier in the course of treatment (or attempted treatment) than others is unclear. In Harlem, for example, where marked social instability was, and continues to be, at the heart of the epidemic, a CDC-designated model program (like programs in New Jersey and San Francisco), under the stewardship of Wafaa El-Sadr, was remarkably successful in ensuring treatment compliance without resorting to detention. Out of more than 500 patients at Harlem Hospital, El-Sadr remembers only a handful of patients requiring long-term detention over a four-year period.[19] Prior rates of failure to complete treatment from this hospital were on the order of 90 percent.[20] Through a uniquely supportive "family-based" model, completion-of-treatment rates have risen to more than 90 percent.[21] Other centers use detention more frequently to encourage compliance. It is unclear whether this illustrates differences in populations being served, in approach to providing tuberculosis services, or in the readiness to resort to detention.

As the number of tuberculosis cases has declined, so too has the number of patients issued orders both for mandatory DOT and detention. The reduction in the number of beds available for detained patients at Goldwater Memorial Hospital reflects this fact. In July 1997 the unit of 29 beds was closed and the smaller overflow unit of 14 beds was made available for detention.

Somewhat surprisingly, both media and civil rights groups have exhibited remarkably little interest in the plight of detained patients. This is probably partly the result of the success of the tuberculosis control program overall and the fact that fewer patients have been detained than some had feared. In addition, leading staff members in several organizations that had shown an interest before the amendments were adopted have left their positions; for example, Robert Levy of the New York Civil

Liberties Union. Of the more than 200 noninfectious cases who have been detained since the amended regulations were adopted, only one has been released following a court hearing.[22] In this case, which was one of the first to be heard following the adoption of the amendments, the court determined that the patient should not be "detained against her will on the mere speculation that eventually the patient will become contagious."[23] Interestingly, it seems that the judge misunderstood the terms "infectious" and "active" tuberculosis, implying that they were one and the same. (Whether this made a difference to the outcome is a moot point.) In all subsequent cases detention has been upheld.

Has representation for patients been sufficiently rigorous? Since April 1993 the Bureau of Tuberculosis Control made the decision to release all but one of the patients discharged from Goldwater's detention unit, and apparently it was not influenced by patients' legal advocates. Indeed, it appears that some patients' legal representatives view their role as supplementary to that of the Department of Health in encouraging patients to see their predicament and enabling them to accept detention. Illustrative of this approach, one patient's attorney commented to me, "Listen, these people have had so many chances before they get here, they're not going to take their stuff." Apparently he explicitly acknowledged that he saw his role as "supportive" of the bureau. My observations suggest that a very comfortable arrangement has developed between the Department of Health and patients' attorneys, which translates into patients only rarely being released from detention by the courts. Several of the city's bureau officials and lawyers concur with this observation. A number of bureau employees have suggested that the checks and balances in the process of detention take place not at the hearings but in the Bureau of Tuberculosis Control, where health officials decide each case carefully and reconsider each one at regular and frequent intervals while each individual is detained. If this is so, then the process of law, specifically appropriate and adequate legal representation, is failing these patients.

LEGAL RESPONSES ELSEWHERE IN THE UNITED STATES

Since the early 1990s New York has detained far more patients with tuberculosis than other cities and states. Indeed, many states have not amended their public health regulations to enable the authorities to detain noninfectious, noncompliant individuals, despite 1993 CDC recommendations.[24] In 1995, when ethicist Ann Alpers and her colleagues from the University of California, San Francisco conducted a 50-state legal survey, only 12 states (California, Delaware, Florida, Maine, Michigan, Minnesota, Montana, New Jersey, New York, Oregon, Rhode Island, and Texas) explicitly authorized public health authorities to detain poorly compliant noninfectious patients. Seven states (Alabama, Connecticut, Indiana, Maryland, Massachusetts, Virginia, and Washington) and the District of Columbia authorized the detention of patients until they no longer pose a threat to the public health.[25] Several states used the New York City amendments as a template on which to base their own local public health regulations. California, in particular, adopted New York's regulations almost verbatim. But there have been problems, not least the lack of adequate facilities. As in several other states, patients in California initially were detained under a criminal code in jails, yet released early in part because it was clear this was an unsuitable environment to encourage a long-term therapeutic response, and also because jails were already overstretched and overpopulated.[26] Other states, such as Texas and Florida, also used jails to detain noncompliant patients, but again, few were detained for long periods for similar reasons. The influence of the New York response, with dedicated facilities and far-reaching civil authority to detain noninfectious patients, and the consequences are still being felt. The number of patients detained long-term in New York dwarfs those detained elsewhere although, as a proportion of patient numbers, other states have higher rates of detention (but almost universally for shorter periods).[27]

In all probability the substantial number of individuals being detained in New York City reflects the nature of the population being served, the fact that adequate facilities exist (as they do now in Massachusetts and Florida), and that the detention procedure is now streamlined. The relatively low overall detention rate (about 1 percent) in New York City reflects the extent of the efforts to which officials, particularly outreach workers, go to ensure compliance in the community. At other sites in the United States detention rates of up to 10 percent have been suggested.[28] Yet, unlike elsewhere in the United States, prolonged detention (i.e., detention until cure) is the rule in New York rather than the exception for most noninfectious individuals who end up detained for poor treatment compliance. Again, this probably reflects the population served, the streamlined nature of the bureau's detention and review process, the lack of vigorous legal representation for patients, and the availability of dedicated facilities. As the tuberculosis rate continues to decline and the city renegotiates its contract (and presumably reduces its support) for care of indigent tuberculosis patients, economies of scale may mean that alternatives to dedicated facilities will have to be considered. As of mid-1999 that situation has not yet arrived.

SOCIAL POLICIES OF THE 1990S

As Robert Koch noted more than a century ago, there is a balance between social conditions and disease, and any response should not be assessed in isolation. Despite the successes of the public health response to the epidemic, other broader social policies introduced in the 1990s (or continued from the 1980s) have the potential to reduce the impact of public health control measures and influence their practical application. Some of these policies may inhibit efforts toward prevention of spread, delay detection of active cases, and delay treatment initiation. Furthermore, some policies may further alienate patients and aggravate treatment compliance problems. The following sections briefly describe some of the changes that have occurred since the public health response to the epidemic took place and analyze their potential impact on public health efforts to control tuberculosis.

HEALTHCARE REFORM

In the past decade the healthcare delivery system in the United States has changed substantially from a fee-for-service to capitation-based system, from independent medical practitioners to managed-care organizations, from nominally "not-for-profit" institutions to a sector in which for-profit providers and institutions are expanding their market share considerably. President Clinton's insurance plan, whereby individuals could enroll in one of three plans (indemnity with maximum choice, managed care with the opportunity to step outside the system, and restricted managed care) failed to get support. Even if it had been implemented successfully, millions still would have remained without healthcare coverage, a fact often neglected or ignored. As the United States does not have a national universal healthcare plan, millions currently receive poor healthcare. Between 1991 and 1996 the uninsured proportion of the population increased from 15.9 percent to 17.6 percent, and New York State caught up to and exceeded the national average in failing to provide adequate healthcare coverage. In 1991, 13.9 percent of New Yorkers had no health insurance, but by 1996 the figure stood at 19.1 percent, more than 3 million individuals. Almost 40 percent of adults in the state in families with incomes below 200 percent of the poverty level were uninsured in 1996. In the city the figures were worse still: 28 percent of city residents are uninsured.[29]

Ensuring healthcare quality for those covered by health maintenance organizations (HMOs), rather than expanding coverage, is now the focus of political attention. Those covered by Medicaid (considerably fewer than the number eligible) are increasingly enrolling in HMOs, which in some cases are a distinct improvement on earlier times. The plans offer improved access to primary care, and those with coverage are now being encouraged to make use of preventive medical care rather than, as in the past, being actively dissuaded from seeking healthcare. But deceptive marketing and enrollment practices, underservice, inadequate access to specialty care, and low-quality care (not to mention outright fraud) still pervade HMOs. But the system is in a state of flux. Recently several HMOs have pulled out of Medicaid managed care because of concerns over cost. Whichever system eventually caters to those with Medicaid, some coverage, however inadequate, will be provided. Those without any coverage, however, are largely ignored, and a universal healthcare system seems farther away than ever. Indeed, despite the number of Americans without healthcare insurance, in 1999 neither the Republicans nor the Democrats appear to view *universal* healthcare as a "critical" issue.

HOMELESSNESS AND HOUSING

Overcrowding, already a substantial problem in the early 1990s, has become worse. The proportion of individuals living in the city in severely crowded renter households (an average of more than 1.5 persons per room) increased such that in 1996, it represented 3.5 percent of rented accommodation. This has been the consequence of several policy decisions.

Federal funding for programs for the elderly and disabled from the U.S. Department of Housing and Urban Development (HUD) was cut from $24.97 billion in 1992 to $19.5 billion in 1997. Federal spending on Incremental Section 8, a support program to assist low-income households to afford private rents, fell from $2.786 billion to zero. With this the expansion of public housing slowed. The availability of fewer affordable housing units has aggravated overcrowding and/or homelessness. Increasing the costs for low-income families, the City Rent Stabilization Guidelines Board increased rents and imposed a levy of $25 on properties renting below $400. Public construction of new homes declined in the 1990s under Mayor Giuliani's stewardship. In 1997 construction was planned for just over 7,000 units, 25 percent fewer than annually during the Dinkins era, and the number of apartments constructed for the homeless fell by 50 percent between 1996 and 1997, to under 600.[30]

By 1996 homelessness had not been eased. During the 1990s the city experienced a 9 percent increase in the number of homeless children under ten years old. Yet welfare reform, discussed next, has not produced a surge in homelessness that many expected. This fact may be related in part to the strength of the economy (unemployment is at a 25-year low), and for a while, at least, most "can survive on the patchwork help of family and friends."[31] But no one knows how long this can continue or what the implications of a faltering economy may have on homelessness rates.

WELFARE REFORM

On August 22, 1996, President Clinton signed the Personal Responsibility and Work Opportunity Reconciliation Act of 1996 (PRA), establishing new welfare policies. With the enactment of the PRA, the Aid to Families with Dependent Children (AFDC) program, a 61-year-old federal guarantee of income to needy families, ceased to exist. It was replaced by the Temporary Assistance for Needy Families (TANF) program. PRA creates or regulates two separate block grants in addition to TANF (one for social services and one for child care), and states have much greater flexibility to channel money through these block grants, redirecting, if they so wish, money to programs for the less needy. Although TANF gives block grants to states for poverty-related programs, and the amount is set at the level the state was receiving for AFDC in 1994 (and increased at 1 percent per year), states can reduce their own poverty-directed contributions by up to 25 percent. In other words, nationally, between 1997 and 2002, $40 billion of state funds could be withdrawn or redirected away from antipoverty programs (in addition to federal cuts).

Besides giving states greater flexibility in determining how to spend funds on poverty, TANF is significantly different from AFDC in one other important respect: Eligibility for TANF support is time-limited. That is, aid is available to any family for a maximum of 60 months. Although welfare rolls have fallen substantially as the economy has expanded, and people are eager to "store up" their benefit for worse days ahead, it is unclear whether the savings are being redirected toward education and skills building to maintain and expand opportunities for the poor. New York's governor and the city's mayor were, in 1998, vying to see who would appear more fiscally conservative, with each advocating income tax reductions and further reductions in public service support. Certainly strong markets have created opportunities, even for the least skilled but it is not clear whether those leaving the welfare rolls are becoming employed, and, if they are, whether that employment is leading to further training and improvements in future job opportunities, or is merely in a poorly paying job that offers little opportunity for advancement and perhaps a return to unemployment. In New York City it is estimated that there will be too few jobs for job-seekers. If every new job was given to a welfare recipient, it would take an estimated 21 years for all recipients to be absorbed into the economy.[32] Supporting this contention the *New York Times* found that the majority of the 8,000 women who had completed the city's four week "job-readiness club" "pounded the pavement with resumes and newly fired dreams" but most failed to find work.[33] By the end of 1997 national evidence suggested that only about half of those leaving the welfare rolls were becoming employed and that, although the number of workers was rising, "so is the number of families with neither benefits nor jobs."[34] In New York City Mayor Giuliani has declined to track welfare recipients, so it is impossible to determine how many are getting jobs. What will happen to those who stay on welfare or those who are incapable of holding down a job? New York proportionately has more than the national average of those on welfare long-term. Pressures on states to push these individuals into work will become greater (in order to not dip into state funds) as they exceed the five-year federal time limit on welfare receipt. Will states support these individuals with their own funds (creating greater burdens on some states and their tax payers), or will they end up in jails, again another expensive alternative or, most likely, ignored and homeless, at least for a time? One of the PRA's main sponsors warned of future difficulties when he commented, "It's going to get tougher, no doubt."[35] Yet few states, including New York, are putting money aside for rainier days.

As most legal immigrants are exempt from welfare support in their first five years, the threat of a rising immigrant homeless population is very real. In November 1994 California voters approved overwhelmingly Proposition 187, which denied publicly funded healthcare to illegal immigrants. (The courts subsequently denied the proposition's implementation.) Under the new welfare reforms, illegal immigrants are ineligible for any federal benefits except emergency, noncash services, such as soup kitchens and emergency medical treatment. With increasing numbers of immigrants to the United States being diagnosed with tuberculosis, the consequences of poor healthcare access may be substantial, as patients either avoid or delay seeking treatment. It is worth remembering that in New York City in 1997, more than 65 percent of the 50,000 patients for whom the Bureau of Tuberculosis Control provided services were foreign born.[36] With regard to the California vote, there were calls by doctors to consider popular sentiments regarding the provision of nonemergency care to illegal immigrants. Two notable tuberculosis experts, Michael Iseman and Jeffrey Starke, commented, for example, that "Although it is emotionally easy to justify circumventing regulations that limit care, we risk the loss of public confidence if we ignore the burgeoning, sometimes passionate sentiments of our fellow citizens." These authors advocated "steps . . . be taken at our borders to curtail the influx of illegal immigrants."[37] Others reflected that "physicians may have a moral duty to provide care to patients in need, regardless of their financial or citizenship status."[38] Obviously exempting some residents from healthcare, particularly when they are the most vulnerable and needy, is ethically questionable. Not only is the Hippocratic oath brought into question, but legislators' overeagerness to pander to public sentiments and constrain spending on those who are "undeserving" threatens the public health.

Under the PRA, states have the option to continue or deny Medicaid to legal immigrants. In New York coverage has been continued for immigrants who were already in the country before the date PRA was enacted (August 22, 1996). Immigrants arriving after that date are ineligible for Medicaid for five years but are eligible for emergency Medicaid. Illegal immigrants in New York are eligible only for emergency programs *and* for treatment of communicable diseases. How patients know they have a communicable disease before seeking care, however, is not made clear. In 1997 more than two-thirds of patients provided for by the bureau were without Medicaid or any other healthcare insurance, and illegal immigrants undoubtedly will delay seeking care, which will prolong the time they are infectious and threaten the public health, as early reports are suggesting.[39] Fear of being reported to the authorities will make follow-up considerably more onerous for public health officials, increase alienation, and compromise compliance. Public anxiety may rise and be focused once again on the "undeserving" consumptive. The recent past may mirror the near future.

INEQUALITY

Through the mid- to late 1990s, the U.S. economy boomed. In 1998 national unemployment was lower than it had been for a quarter of a century. Jobs were available. Since 1983 the economy produced nearly 2 million jobs a year, and between 1993 and 1997, 10 million new jobs were generated nationally. The national unemployment rate has fallen to below 5 percent. Many of those employed have benefited from the economy's growth including many of the poorest, most ill educated, and least skilled. Yet the benefits of the economic boom have been felt, as always, unequally.

The gap between the wealthy and poor is wider than ever. By 1994 the top 1 percent of the national population was earning as much after taxes as the bottom 35 percent (a 72 percent increase since 1977, nearly eight times the average gain), and tax legislation introduced in August 1997 exacerbated this disparity.[40] By 1996 only the top fifth of the population had an average income above prerecession levels of the early 1990s. The top 20 percent of households received as much as the remaining 80 percent of the population combined, the highest ratio since the Census Bureau began collecting that data 30 years earlier (1994 showed the same figure).[41] And New York continues to lead the field in income inequality. By the mid-1990s the average income of the poorest fifth of families in the state was $9,250, a *drop* of $270 from the mid-1980s. During this period the richest increased their income by $16,460, to $117,500.[42] Moreover, racial differences in income inequality are marked in New York City. Whereas non-Hispanic white family incomes had recovered by 1995 to 1990 levels (median $45,194), black family incomes continued to fall (from median $28,171 to $22,950).[43]

The trend in income disparity between those who are better educated and those who are not has continued. Between 1980 and 1996, while earnings of college graduates rose by 12 percent, the median wage of those with only a high school diploma fell by 6 percent. Moreover, beyond income, benefits (which earlier were perceived as an important equalizer) for workers have been spread unequally, widening the inequality gap for those employed. For example, health insurance, paid vacation leave, and pension plans are all offered to workers at the top of the pay scale, but most at the bottom do not benefit. In 1996 more than 80 percent of workers received paid holidays. Less than 10 percent of those in the bottom 10 percent did. Seventy percent of workers have pension plans, yet less than 10 percent of those at the bottom can count on employer-financed retirement plans. The story is the same with health insurance.[44] And housing. Rent inflation in the 1990s, which has outstripped wage increases, means more income is being spent on housing, and "disposable" income is shrinking. This has hit the poor hardest, compounded income disparity, and threatens to increase the homeless population. Inequalities are greater, therefore, than those obvious from data on income alone suggest. As an economist from the University of Chicago noted, "Unskilled workers get the short end of the stick—and it's getting shorter."[45] The inequalities of the 1980s have been perpetuated and threaten to grow further.

POVERTY

Poverty levels improved nationally since 1993, as would be expected with falling unemployment. Yet, when compared to 1989, when unemployment rates were equivalent, and the economy in 1996 was stronger than 1989, poverty rates are higher, at 13.7 percent compared to 13.1 percent.[46] Likewise, in New York City, poverty rates have fallen since 1993 but remain higher than during the similar period of economic growth of the late 1980s, and persist at about double the national average. Furthermore, extreme poverty is still prevalent. Seventy-five percent of the city's poor residents live in extreme poverty (subsisting on less than 75 percent of the poverty level). Unemployment has fallen in the city but, unlike earlier decades, remains substantially higher than national rates. Moreover, unemployment in young men remains high. For example, in a survey conducted in March 1996, 22.9 percent of New York City men aged between 25 and 44 were jobless (71 percent higher than joblessness in this age group as a whole in the nation).[47]

Poverty in the city continues to affect minorities, female-headed families, and children disproportionately. The poverty rate in 1995 among blacks was 35.2 percent and among Hispanics, 42.2 percent. Fifty-seven percent of families headed by women at this time were living in poverty. Just over 40 percent of all New York City's children live in poverty, and more than 70 percent of those who live with only their mother do so.[48]

Overall in New York then, poverty and extreme poverty are still prevalent and concentrated particularly in minority women and children. Although unemployment has fallen, it remains higher than the national average and structurally different with almost no opportunity to escape for the dispossessed, a departure from earlier economic cycles. This bodes poorly for the future. Substantial numbers of individuals have been unable to take advantage of the economic upturn, and social exclusion remains a potent ingredient in New York's cultural makeup.

CONCLUSION

New York City's public health response to the chaos of the tuberculosis epidemic has undoubtedly been successful. Tuberculosis rates have fallen more rapidly than anyone would have predicted, rates of MDRTB have declined substantially, and the increases in childhood tuberculosis have been reversed. Yet many social policies have the potential to stymie these efforts. The economic expansion that the United States is enjoying obscures explicit recognition of this fact. The seeds that caused the tuberculosis epidemic and necessitated such harsh measures for some individuals are still present and, some would say, are potentially being made worse. The pressures on city and state public purses will increase still further as the federal time limit for welfare support approaches, and the consequences may be dire if economic slowdown occurs, as it surely will at some point. Then, once again, the disaffected population will grow, the homeless population will increase, civil distrust will rise, and calls for improved control of crime and public health will be raised. Jail populations will continue to swell, and the strain on the public purse will cause further voter alienation. Once again public health authorities will be under pressure to "do something," and they will request further support from federal sources. The cycle will repeat, unless there is political will to break the mold and the current budget surplus is used to improve education, create real job opportunities, eradicate institutionalized inequities, and remedy the structural causes of social exclusion. Calls to maintain support of the public health infrastructure will be heard, and probably heeded, at least in the short term. But once again public health authorities will have to respond to the wave of disaffection, distrust, and poverty that shall surely bring, in its wake, more tuberculosis. The opportunity to act positively for the long-term may not exist in the future.

A Real Threat to Public Health?

Fear of harm ought to be proportional not merely to the gravity of the harm, but also to the probability of the event.

—Blaise Pascal, *La logique, ou l'art de penser,* 1662

To support the strategy of expanded directly observed therapy, New York City health codes were amended to give the commissioner of health the authority to mandate DOT and, as a last resort, to detain both infectious and noninfectious individuals with tuberculosis who could not be relied upon to comply with treatment.[1] In increasing its authority to detain noninfectious individuals with tuberculosis, the New York City Department of Health argued that an assessment of aggregate risk posed by these patients was important because "emphasis must be placed on the cumulative or likely risk to the public health created by noncompliance with tuberculosis treatment in a number of persons or by a single individual over time." The department recognized that any one individual noncompliant patient may only pose a "small risk directly to the public" but argued that the risk increases if many patients fail to comply with treatment. They further argued that "over time, it is likely that they will pose a very serious threat to large segments of the public."[2] This represented a fundamental shift in officials' authority to include measures directed toward noninfectious recalcitrant patients. Since the amended regulations were adopted in

April 1993, more than 200 noninfectious individuals have been detained by the city, some for considerable periods of time.

At the time the amended regulations were adopted, concern both from civil libertarians and city officials was largely focused on "due process" protections with an emphasis on the use of less restrictive alternatives to detention. Both sides broadly accepted the constitutional and ethical principles underlying the justification for detention of "recalcitrant" individuals, and little distinction was made between whether they were infectious or noninfectious.[3] Although the primary goal was the reduction of the threat to public health, little attention, particularly by those opposing the regulatory changes, was paid to the uncertainty regarding the risk of relapse or the actual magnitude of the threat posed by noninfectious, poorly compliant individuals. David Rothman, chairman of the New York Academy of Medicine Committee on Single Disease Institutions for Tuberculosis, voiced the assumption at the heart of the debate when he stated: "Were it not for the graveness of the danger of contagion and resistant organisms, none of this program [of detention] would pass legal scrutiny or gain the endorsement of those who are familiar with the history of confinement or who have a commitment to civil libertarian traditions."[4]

Do poorly compliant noninfectious individuals in fact pose "a significant risk to the health or safety of others" and was the city's reaction not merely a response to "irrational fears, speculation, stereotypes, or pernicious mythologies"?[5] This chapter provides an objective assessment of the threat posed by noninfectious individuals and explores other factors that may have influenced the interpretation of these data and hence led to a more subjective assessment and perhaps less reliable measure of the threat posed by "recalcitrant" individuals. Surprisingly, the concept of risk, or public health threat, posed by noninfectious individuals received scant attention as the amendments were drawn up. But an understanding of risk is crucial to assessing the policy decisions.[6] As Howard Leichter, a professor of political science, wrote in his book *Free to Be Foolish* "Among the most basic questions that must be addressed before the public and policymakers can and should endorse regulation of personal behavior in the name of health promotion is the degree of certainty linking a particular life-style practice to a health harm."[7] So what threat did poorly compliant, noninfectious individuals with tuberculosis pose?

HOW INFECTIOUS IS TUBERCULOSIS?

There are large gaps in our understanding of the transmission dynamics of tuberculosis, including measures that determine exposure to the causative organism, *Mycobacterium tuberculosis,* susceptibility to disease, infectiousness of a person, and a detailed understanding of the factors that influence these variables. Studies have largely relied on the tuberculin skin test, a measure of the person's immune response to mycobacterial protein and therefore an indicator of earlier exposure, but this test is both unreliable and difficult to interpret.[8] Much of what is accepted dogmatically with regard to the transmissibility of tuberculosis is in fact "wishful thinking based on a few scant facts."[9]

In some important experiments in the 1950s, Richard Riley, of Johns Hopkins University, and his coworkers demonstrated and clarified both the airborne nature of tuberculosis transmission and established that one organism of *M. tuberculosis* in 11,000 cubic feet of air was sufficient to cause infection in guinea pigs.[10] In these experiments, air from a tuberculosis ward was channeled into exposure chambers where guinea pigs were housed and the incidence of positive tuberculin reactors assessed. It is unclear, however, whether humans are equally susceptible.

Riley and coworkers also showed that the infectivity of any patient varies considerably, even when similar clinical characteristics were present.[11] Factors determining the infectiousness of any case include the smear status (i.e., whether organisms can be seen microscopically on sputum samples), treatment status, and frequency of cough.[12] Like the tuberculin test, smear status is an important diagnostic tool but, again like the tuberculin test, a blunt tool. The data suggesting that smear-positive cases are infectious, however, are consistent. Community-based studies, where the tuberculin status of a given community is ascertained and all cases of pulmonary tuberculosis identified (and the tuberculin reactivity in young children is used to define transmission rates), show that household contacts of smear-positive individuals have rates of tuberculin positivity 30 to 50 percent above those of age-matched controls. Contacts of smear-negative, culture-positive cases show rates only about 5 percent above controls.[13] It has been estimated that approximately one secondary active case of tuberculosis arises each month from one untreated smear-positive case.[14] In support of the impact of smear status on infectiousness, nosocomial outbreaks have been interrupted by isolating smear-positive cases. A further confounding problem in tuberculosis control, however, is the question of "efficient disseminators." It may be that some individuals are able to expose contacts to *M. tuberculosis* more readily than others, but determining who these individuals are before they do so is not yet possible.[15] Moreover, some strains of *M. tuberculosis* may be more easily transmitted, or infectiousness, although not of great magnitude, may be present for years.[16] Smear status of source patients and genetic variability in human susceptibility appear to influence progression to disease in contacts. Tuberculosis is more common, for example, among tuberculin-positive contacts of smear-positive cases than among tuberculin-positive contacts of smear-negative source cases, which suggests that the magnitude of the exposure plays a role in disease development.[17] It is clear, therefore, that although outbreaks have originated from smear-negative source cases, smear-negative individuals are considerably less infectious than smear-positive ones and probably do not pose a significant threat to the public;[18] if certain smear-negative individuals do pose such a threat, identifying them is, at present, impossible.

Host factors may play a part. Disease has been reported to be more severe in blacks compared to whites, and recent evidence suggests that several polymorphisms in a gene (the NRAMP1 gene), which is important in killing intracellular pathogens such as *M. tuberculosis,* may confer increased susceptibility to tuberculosis, at least in some populations.[19]

The relative contagiousness of drug-resistant strains in comparison to drug-susceptible strains is unknown. It has been shown, however, from isolates collected in New York City between January 1990 and August 1993 that more than one-third of all multidrug-resistant tuberculosis cases had identical or nearly identical restriction fragment length polymorphism (RFLP) patterns (i.e., DNA fingerprint analysis), indicating clustering. Furthermore, the clustered cases in this outbreak, which involved 11 hospitals, represented nearly a quarter of patients with MDRTB in the United States over the period studied. At least 86 percent of patients were HIV infected.[20] This suggests that the acquisition of drug resistance (at least to some drugs), while it may interfere with infectiousness of tuberculosis, does not do so dramatically. Indeed, in cases of drug-resistant tuberculosis, the infectious period from any source patient may be extended, increasing the opportunity for more contacts to be exposed and infected.

HIV certainly plays an important role in increasing the risk of progression to disease following exposure, and it may be important in transmission with those whose immune system is relatively unimpaired being better transmitters. However, it probably plays no part in increasing the risk of exposure, other than through associated sociodemographic factors such as hospitalization, prison, poverty, drug use, and overcrowding.[21]

Thus, with our current knowledge, determining the infectiousness and future infectiousness of any individual with tuberculosis is an uncertain science. Yet some facts are clear. Infectiousness is considerably increased in patients who have respiratory disease and are smear positive, and HIV contributes substantially to the risk of disease development following infection with *M. tuberculosis*. We also know that as treatment continues the risk of relapse falls.

TREATMENT COMPLIANCE, RELAPSE, AND DRUG RESISTANCE

One of the principal aims of New York City's Department of Health from 1992 onwards was to increase treatment compliance and completion-of-treatment rates to prevent both further spread of tuberculosis and the development of acquired resistance.

Why does drug resistance occur? Mathematical probability. The bacterial population in cavitary pulmonary tuberculosis (i.e., disease affecting the lungs and producing necrotic holes) is estimated at between 10^7 to 10^9 organisms, and spontaneous mutations leading to drug resistance occur with a frequency of approximately 1 in 10^6 to 10^8 replications, depending on the drug.[22] Given these odds, there is a high probability that resistance to a single drug is present even before treatment begins, and then of mutations emerging and becoming predominant due to selection pressure if single-agent therapy is used. Sites for resistance are chromosomally located and are not linked; therefore, the likelihood of an organism spontaneously developing resistance to two agents falls substantially and may be on the order of only 1 in 10^{14}. Use of at least two drugs to which the organism is sensitive, therefore, means that the probability of resistance developing becomes negligible, but these two drugs need to be taken together, not sequentially.

In the era before AIDS, 25 percent of those with untreated pulmonary tuberculosis continued to shed mycobacteria during the fifth year of follow-up.[23] However, with conventional treatment over six months using four drugs (isoniazid, rifampin, ethambutol, and pyrazinamide for the initial phase, and rifampin and isoniazid alone for the continuation phase), very few relapses (on the order of 1 percent at two years and 3 percent at five years) occur if there is no initial drug resistance.[24] If short-course chemotherapy, as it is termed, is reduced to four months, relapse rates are substantially higher (on the order of 13 percent at two years), as they are also with three- and two-month regimens.[25] Since it takes, on average, eight weeks to convert from smear positive to smear negative, many patients will need to undergo at least two months of treatment before being deemed noninfectious. (However, actual infectiousness, rather than a change in smear status, undoubtedly declines rapidly after the introduction of treatment.)[26] From clinical trials, the probability of relapse (determined without the benefit of confirmation by molecular techniques such as RFLP typing) can be quantifiably estimated from the duration of treatment given. However, when treatment is erratic, when only some drugs are taken but not others, and when there is primary or acquired drug resistance at the commencement of treatment (or retreatment), estimating the risk of relapse and the possibility that further drug resistance has developed is, in practice, almost impossible. In day-to-day clinical practice (in cases where HIV prevalence is not sizable), when little supervision occurs, relapse rates on the order of 20 percent may be seen over several years.[27] In other settings, such as clinical trials, relapse rates are substantially lower, suggesting that in routine clinical practice noncompliance may be a frequent event, as it is in most chronic conditions.

Coexistent HIV infection probably increases the risk of relapse when treatment is incomplete. For example, in one study approximately one-quarter of those patients (who were at high risk of HIV infection) who failed to complete three months of treatment apparently relapsed within one year, a substantial increase above the expected rate of relapse of 13 percent or so if all patients had been HIV negative (assuming they had received at least two months of treatment).[28] Some uncertainty surrounds the influence of HIV on relapse rates, however. First, most reports of relapse in this population have been determined clinically (without the benefit of confirmation by molecular techniques); and second, most HIV-infected individuals with tuberculosis from New York City lived in areas of high endemicity for tuberculosis. This fact may have increased the risk of reexposure, which, with rapid progression to active disease, would simulate relapse. Finally, since many HIV-infected patients who develop tuberculosis are unaware of their HIV status, and many are not offered testing, the picture becomes quite confusing.

How should society respond when the public health risks posed by any individual recalcitrant patient may be small and uncertain? And what is the evidence that isolation is effective at reducing the public health threat?

SEGREGATION AND TUBERCULOSIS CONTROL

PRE–ANTIMICROBIAL ERA

In the *pre*–antibiotic era, up to the 1940s, inpatient care for individuals with tuberculosis served a number of purposes. At that time treatment consisted only of bedrest and nutritional support (with surgery occasionally), measures from which Edward Livingston Trudeau's early animal experiments had provided a template.[29] (Trudeau showed in the 1880s that rabbits with tuberculosis that were well cared for survived, whereas those that were neglected died.) Recovery rates in individuals with mild disease were good.[30] In addition, these facilities isolated infectious individuals from the community for prolonged periods, sometimes years, and, it has been argued, this measure protected the public health. Interestingly, at this time (around the turn of the century) concern over the perceived threat to the general public grew and coercive measures toward uncooperative patients were implemented, as noted in chapter 2. These recalcitrant individuals, or "rounders," who drifted in and out of hospitals were once described as "homeless, friendless, dependent, dissipated and vicious consumptives" and were then, as now, perceived as "likely to be most dangerous to the community."[31]

Thomas McKeown, professor of Social Medicine at Birmingham, England, and others have suggested that the decline in tuberculosis rates in the pre–antibiotic era was secondary to broad increases in the standard of living and, in particular, in improvements in nutrition; they believe that isolation and other narrowly focused public health measures had little impact.[32] Others believe that targeted interventions, including the isolation of patients, played an important role in the reduction of tuberculosis rates.[33] Historians Amy Fairchild and Gerald Oppenheimer of Columbia University have reviewed both sides of the debate recently.[34] Quantitative supportive evidence does not to enable a clear determination of the influence of improvements in social conditions on tuberculosis rates above those of specific interventions. For example, in New York City, despite the increase in isolation of individuals with tuberculosis coinciding with the fall in tuberculosis rates, there is considerable uncertainty over whether this is just cause and effect. First, there were too few facilities. For example, in 1919 only 14 percent of the city's 32,048 registered cases were institutionalized. Second, individuals frequently took their own discharge, so isolation from the wider public was at best erratic. Last, and in this context perhaps most important, the vast majority of the public would already have been exposed to and infected by *M. tuberculosis*. For example, in 1907, 60 percent of children had been infected in urban areas.[35] As commentators of the time pointed out, "Infection, of itself, is relatively unimportant. The problem of preventing the outbreak of frank disease in the legions of the infected is the crux of the program of prevention."[36] When the majority of the population has already been exposed, isolating even infectious patients may serve little purpose.

Others have suggested that isolation may have had a more profound effect. A natural experiment, it has been proposed, occurred toward the end of the nineteenth century in the United Kingdom. While social conditions were improving during this time in Ireland, England, Wales, and Scotland, tuberculosis mortality rates were declining everywhere but in Ireland. In England, Wales, and Scotland, the ill poor, who would most likely have been those suffering from tuberculosis, often were sent to Poor Law infirmaries and workhouses. That is, they were segregated from friends, family, and neighbors. In Ireland, however, relief was provided at home. Increased segregation in Britain may have resulted in a reduction in the probability of transmission and consequent disease and mortality.[37] In further support of the benefits of segregation, it has been claimed that a steeper decline in tuberculosis rates occurred when segregation was widely used.[38] Muddying the waters further, however, other specific interventions also may have been influential, and perhaps to a greater degree, in the decline of tuberculosis rates. With the introduction of pasteurization, for example, childhood tuberculosis rates, most especially of extrapulmonary disease, fell dramatically through a reduction in transmission of *Mycobacterium bovis* through milk.[39]

In all probability, tuberculosis rates fell in the pre–antibiotic era for a variety of reasons, with improved social conditions (reduced overcrowding, better ventilation, improved nutrition), segregation and the sanatoria movement, and pasteurization all playing a part. A reliable estimate of the magnitude of the influence that each factor had on the trend cannot be made.

POST–ANTIMICROBIAL ERA

Is there evidence that isolation of infectious individuals in the *post*–antibiotic era is effective, when a much lower percentage of the urban population has been exposed to the disease? Again, there are few data on which to make a judgment. Isolation or segregation of infectious patients has been used as a public health tool only infrequently since effective antibiotics were introduced. With so few cases being isolated, attempting to draw any meaningful inferences is difficult.

One influential study from the antibiotic era has colored our views regarding family members' exposure risk and weakened arguments for isolation of infectious individuals from their family at the commencement of treatment.[40] This study showed that removing infectious individuals from their homes has little impact on contacts subsequently being exposed to, or developing, tuberculosis. The study, conducted over five years, assessed "attack rates" of tuberculosis in close family contacts of source cases. Source cases were randomly assigned to receive therapy at home or in a sanatorium. Contacts were followed up with tuberculin skin tests and chest radiography. There were no differences in tuberculin conversion rates or tuberculosis rates between contacts of either group, suggesting that no benefits were gained from isolation. This study was, however, performed in the 1950s in Madras, India, an area highly endemic for tuberculosis. It would be unwise to extrapolate from these data the conclusion that segregation in low-prevalence areas would not result in reduced transmission from infectious patients and ultimately decreased disease. Yet clinical practice in the West is such that infectious individuals are frequently quarantined at home with their family (who are assumed to have been exposed) until they are deemed no longer infectious.

Although our understanding of the transmission dynamics of tuberculosis is far from complete, what is clear is that tuberculosis is an airborne pathogen and that environmental changes can hinder its spread. What is also clear is that cases of nonpulmonary tuberculosis and smear-negative pulmonary tuberculosis are considerably less infectious than smear-positive pulmonary tuberculosis. Individuals with extrapulmonary and smear-negative pulmonary tuberculosis, by and large, do not "imminently" threaten the public health (although recent research suggests a sizable minority of patients with tuberculosis acquired the infection from a smear-negative source patient).[41] On an individual basis, it is difficult to predict what risk of relapse individuals who are poorly compliant with treatment face and what chance they will relapse with a drug-resistant strain. Faced with these uncertainties, a sizable proportion of the population at increased risk of developing tuberculosis if exposed (particularly those with HIV infection), and a need by public health officials to back up less coercive measures, regulations allowing the detention of noninfectious poorly compliant individuals were enacted. In the end, it was a *subjective* decision that was made in response to the *perceived* risk.

THE PERCEPTION OF RISK AND ITS INFLUENCE

The essence of the response of New York City to the recent tuberculosis epidemic was a fear of an epidemic of multidrug-resistant tuberculosis. Kenneth Ong, deputy commissioner of disease intervention, noted as much in a memo to Margaret Hamburg, Commissioner of Health, on October 6, 1992 in which he underlined the following words: "The increasing prevalence of drug resistant tuberculosis is at the heart of the current public health crisis. If the prevalence of resistant tuberculosis continues to rise, effective cost-efficient outpatient therapy for tuberculosis in the entire city of New York will be compromised and could be lost."[42] The response to this fear hinged on enabling or enhancing the prospect that recalcitrant individuals complete therapy, but if they fail to comply, then more coercive measures would be authorized (i.e., people would be detained).

It was widely perceived, and was in large part true, that tuberculosis in New York City during the 1980s and early 1990s affected principally the homeless, alcoholic, drug dependent, and HIV infected. To most people, the fear of developing multidrug-resistant tuberculosis would be, or should be, enough to encourage adherence to treatment. But as Karen Brudney and Jay Dobkin, of Columbia Presbyterian Hospital, have commented: "To a patient dependent on alcohol or drugs or unable to assume continuity of shelter, the importance of taking a pill or keeping a clinic appointment diminishes drastically."[43] That is, many of the most vulnerable people in society have priorities that may be very different from those of others. Risk perception is not merely dependent on the probability of harm and the gravity of that harm, as Blaise Pascal, the great mathematician, noted in the seventeenth century when he wrote the words quoted in the epigraph. It is also value laden. Behavioral psychology and the science of risk evaluation confirm this notion. Individuals make *subjective* decisions based on both their perception of risk and also on the expected utility of the gain. Furthermore, as the psychologist Amos Tversky has commented, "our preferences . . . can be manipulated by changes in the reference points."[44] People are risk averse when given a choice in some settings and turn into risk seekers when offered the same choice in a different setting. Moreover, individuals are more determined to avoid a negative outcome than to pursue a positive outcome.[45] To some extent the acceptance of risk is dependent on whether the risk is imposed or chosen autonomously. Often individuals are more willing to bear greater risks if the choice is of their own volition rather than one made by "experts" or by those in authority. For example, in the ongoing debate over the link between bovine spongiform encephalopathy and Creutzfeldt-Jakob disease in the United Kingdom, those in authority argue that the risks arising from a particular course of action are too high for the public to bear, yet a substantial number of people have argued against this position, suggesting that the risks are so small that they are worth taking.[46] This complex response to risk and perceived risk may help to explain why compliance with drugs is so often poor, particularly if drug regimens are associated with unpleasant side effects, as antituberculosis regimens are. The short-term drawbacks from an imposed action (compliance) are outweighed by the uncertainties of disease progression in the longer term and by the fact that the decision not to adhere is apparently a free, un-imposed choice. Added to this, culturally sensitive health beliefs (e.g., "I can't have tuberculosis, I feel well") may result in responses to illness that are both unpredictable and frequently misunderstood.

As with an individual's perception of risk, so society likewise responds to threats in a value-laden manner. In an attempt to reduce and control costs, industrial assessment of risk frequently pits "experts" against laypeople (the public). And experts frequently are wrong in their determination of risk. Medical examples have included the suggestion that breast irradiation to alleviate mastitis is harmless, as is witnessing atomic bomb tests at close range. Another example, perhaps more pertinent to a discussion on detention and public health threat, is worth contemplating. With regard to commitment of the mentally ill, the expert prediction of dangerousness has been shown to be woefully inadequate.[47] As there is no specific mechanism to guarantee the objectivity of a risk decision, science should guide only by attempting to provide theories that both embody values and are transparent and explicit.[48]

Some have questioned the validity of nonexperts' perceptions of risk, but it has become increasingly clear that the perceptions of "experts" are similarly subjective and dependent on value judgments. Daniel Kahneman and Amos Tversky showed that nearly everyone falls victim to biases in the interpretation of statistical data and that experts frequently misjudge risk, typically falling victim to bias from instances or occurrences that can be brought to mind.[49] So in the response to tuberculosis is the perception of risk heightened, for example, by the familiarity with the concept of multidrug-resistant tuberculosis by those public health officials calling for detention as a public health tool or by an unspoken fear of those individuals (the homeless, drug users, HIV infected) who populate the margins of society? This latter fear has been well illustrated historically, from the "deserving" and "undeserving" poor of yesterday to those suffering "through no fault of their own" today. (The implicit suggestion is that others are suffering because of "fault.") The moral politics this approach encourages has been a cornerstone, often unrecognized, of policy decisions. (This issue is further examined in chapter 7.)

Alternatively, or perhaps in addition, was the perception of threat increased by certain cases, such as that of the immunocompromised prison guard with cancer acquiring MDRTB, or other nosocomial outbreaks, including those involving healthcare workers?[50] Although no "signal" event prompted authorities to respond to the epidemic generally, some cases certainly generated considerable publicity, for example outbreaks in prison settings.[51] Mayor Dinkins responded at the time by allocating substantial sums to build dedicated prison isolation units, which, four years later, were largely empty of tuberculosis cases.[52] Adding to the political equation, public interest in tuberculosis was high. By 1993 ten times more articles in magazines and periodicals were appearing on tuberculosis compared to four or five years earlier.

With regard to regulatory processes, liberals, in the context of public health hazards linked to industry, historically have demanded a reduction in risk to workers and the public. They have argued that, where there is uncertainty, decisions should err on the side of caution and protect those whose lives may be at risk. But "conservative" defenders of minimal regulatory constraints would argue that "science," rather than politics should be the arbiter. However, as Columbia professor Ron Bayer has pointed out, "liberal" advocates, in the scenario of possible exposure to HIV from infected healthcare workers have taken a diametrically opposed view to that which they have traditionally held in relation to industry. That is, "liberals who had in the past argued for the most stringent regulatory protections began to assert that there was no such thing as a risk-free environment."[53] Similarly, those conservative supporters of big business who earlier would have argued for fewer restrictions, in the case of hazardous waste, for example, argued for extreme measures to reduce the risk of exposure to HIV. Senator Jesse Helms (R-NC), for example, in calling for the protection of "innocent victims" from exposure to HIV from infected healthcare workers, said he believed in horsewhipping those who failed to disclose their status.[54] Such role changes are not unique to the United States. In the United Kingdom, Theresa Gorman, a Conservative Member of Parliament, recently argued that the mentally ill who have the "tendency" to murder "should be kept in secure accommodation for the rest of their lives."[55] How this tendency can be measured is unclear. In the case of HIV, an about-face has occurred; liberals who in general sought to protect the public from the remotest risks argued that infected healthcare workers posed such small risks to patients that it was irrational to attempt to regulate for that risk, and conservatives advocated for the elimination of *all* risks to patients from healthcare workers.

But tuberculosis is not AIDS, and, it could be argued, health officials are reverting to type with tuberculosis. They are advocating caution and restraint where there is uncertainty, as they have done historically. Debate requires advocates both for and against changing the response to an ill-defined threat. Many of those who voiced opposition to the proposed New York City Health Code amendments at the public hearing were advocates for those infected with HIV. But the HIV-infected population is the very population most threatened by poorly compliant individuals with tuberculosis.[56] Was the opposition muted, or tempered, by concern for their wider constituency? Did this lack of effective opposition enable public health officials to revert to a more "traditional" public health role, such as seen in the pre-AIDS era? The political, media, and public anxiety regarding tuberculosis certainly meant that public health officials' traditional views were broadly supported.[57]

Political and cultural factors also may be important in the perception of and response to risk. Although experts in both the United Kingdom and the United States evaluate risks to the environment in a similar manner, the process of political accountability differs. In the United States the "police powers" that provide for and protect the public health are not held centrally (by federal government) but locally at state level and are delegated to lower levels of government. So, in New York City the authority to detain individuals who pose a threat to the public health lies with the mayor's appointee, the commissioner of health. It can be argued that this fact increases local political awareness, accountability, and responsiveness in the public health arena. But a potential drawback is that the detachment that may be beneficial in a crisis is not present. Furthermore, there is a public hearing before changes or new regulations are adopted, and comments made at the hearing are addressed publicly. It is unlikely that such a detailed debate regarding the detention of noninfectious individuals would have been heard in the United Kingdom, where regulatory public health policymaking is informal, cooperative, less transparent, and more shielded from public scrutiny.[58]

Societal responses to threats, whether they are environmental hazards or new pathogens, appear largely similar on both sides of the Atlantic, although the policy routes by which they were arrived at may vary considerably. For example, when one looks at the public, professional, and media responses to the risk of occupational transmission of HIV from healthcare workers, or the response to asbestos or cigarette smoking, one sees mainly similarities but also a few differences. On occasions, however, although the debate appears similar, the consequences are more radical in one country. For example, the broad measures to counter exposure to cigarette smoke through passive smoking are similar, but it is unlikely that in the United Kingdom smoking will be forbidden in prisons. The concept of zero tolerance (or complete abstention), in order to reduce risk is a more potent notion in the United States, where the concept of risk elimination is more widely accepted. A paradox is seen with regard to gun control. Following the tragedy in Dunblane, Scotland, where several young children were shot, calls for stricter gun control laws were successful; in the United States, despite a large number of shootings in schools recently, measures such as the banning of handguns are politically unattractive, partly because of the power of the gun lobby but also because the historical and cultural framework makes such an approach politically unappealing.

Policy debates may be more immoderate in one country than another with public health officials and politicians "criminalizing" those who pose a public health threat, but the consequences are often similar. Coercive public health measures have not, however, been a major feature in tuberculosis control programs outside the United States yet. In the United Kingdom, for example, legislation allows for the detention of an individual with a notifiable disease who is a threat to others, but this legislation is rarely used.[59] Moreover, there is no legislation to detain an individual who may become a threat in the future.[60] Whether this will remain so if rates of tuberculosis, and particularly rates of drug-resistant tuberculosis, continue to rise is unclear. Indeed, there are rumblings from the British Department of Health suggesting the Public Health (Control of Infection) Act 1984 should be amended or revised to take account of noncompliant individuals. Despite the legal uncertainty of the moves, patients have been issued detention orders for long periods recently.[61]

Where risk is uncertain, some other European countries respond in a manner different from the United States. For example, Norwegians tend to disregard a threat of uncertain magnitude whereas Americans are more demanding of action.[62] However, if the source of threat is an increase in "delinquent" homeless drug addicts, the response, even given America's greater enthusiasm for distinguishing morally between the "deserving" and the "undeserving," may be very similar across Europe to that which occurred in New York City.

With tuberculosis, where RFLP typing provides a mechanism to determine clustering, it might be expected that concerns over litigation would have encouraged U.S. health officials to respond more aggressively. This may have been a factor in encouraging the city to respond to the epidemic, but interestingly, where nosocomial outbreaks resulted in HIV positive individuals acquiring and developing MDRTB, litigation has been more noticeable in the United Kingdom. Two cases recently have been settled out of court for substantial sums, and other cases are ongoing. Perhaps this has been due to greater awareness by British patients (of both the New York City epidemic and nosocomial spread), the increased use of molecular typing techniques (and hence evidence of clustering and in-hospital errors), or because patients have survived long enough to mount a case. An alternative explanation may simply be that those infected in the United Kingdom were middle class, more articulate, and aware that infection control errors had been made.

Thus the response to a public health threat is not simply a response to the probability of a potential event occurring or the magnitude of that event; it is influenced by many subtle (and some not so subtle) individual, societal, and cultural forces. The response by public health officials in New York City to the tuberculosis epidemic, and in particular to recalcitrant noncompliant patients, illustrated many of these forces.

POLICY IMPLICATIONS

How can any coercive public health policy, which by necessity focuses on a disenfranchised group of individuals whose voice may not be heard in policy debates, be as equitable and as fair as possible? Clearly the burden of proof should be more demanding when the consequences of regulation include detention than when only economic penalties follow misdeeds.[63] Furthermore, it must be recognized that, when people feel threatened, they focus inappropriately on external sources, such as stereotyped minorities, and blame them, rather than assessing other threats that are perhaps closer to home (e.g., their hobby of hang-gliding, or smoking, etc.).[64]

One must be clear and explicit about what our goal is. When coercion was used in the South Asia smallpox campaign, the goal was eradication, not control. Although the campaign was successful, concerns have been raised that some of the stringent measures used may hinder future public health campaigns.[65] Most current tuberculosis programs are aimed at control, not eradication, and as a consequence the degree of coercion warranted, if it is at all, should be less. Furthermore, if ongoing cooperation is required for control, the fact that the use of coercion actually may be counterproductive should be considered.

In technological risk assessment, experts frequently overlook many "pathways to disaster"; and there is little reason to believe public health decision making is not equally prone to errors.[66] Perhaps lessons can be learned from the errors of experts that can guide future policy. An attempt should be made to better quantify the threat posed by individuals, both infectious and noninfectious, with tuberculosis. Despite the World Health Organization's assertion that "Everyone who breathes air, from Wall Street to the Great Wall of China, needs to worry about this risk," the risks to all are not equal. For example, those using homeless shelters, when beds were spaced eighteen inches apart and HIV prevalence was high, were obviously at greater risk of exposure compared to those in the leafy suburbs. Policy decisions should involve assessments that are both individualized, as required by law, and weighted to account for expert views on probabilities (and perhaps further weighted on the basis of past predictive success), on economic calculations, and on ethical analysis. Risk assessment must be based on complex theoretical analyses such as fault trees (weighting the potential advantages and disadvantages of different scenarios) rather than direct experience, and it must be recognized explicitly that despite an appearance of objectivity, these analyses will include a large component of judgment. Experts, relying on educated intuition, must determine the structure of the problem, the consequences to be considered, and the importance of the various branches of the fault tree.[67] Furthermore, the public and decision makers should evaluate whether the consequences of policy decisions are similar to or different from those predicted. This transparency of policy analysis may be more readily achieved in some cultures than in others; this fact also needs to be recognized if policies are to be transposed effectively from culture to culture.

An approach to understanding tuberculosis risk must, therefore, define the risk of an event occurring (e.g., the transmission of tuberculosis), determine the gravity of that event, weigh different available measures to be taken, and adjust that perception of risk over time both as understanding improves and as circumstances change. As new information is made available, and as understanding of the perceived threats improves or changes, one's view of the probabilities of potential events occurring must be altered. In addition, the legislative and regulatory approach to coercive public health measures should be responsive to changing perceptions of risk and encourage swift modifications of public health measures.

CONCLUSION

In the early 1990s, given the circumstances (and the perception thereof), the uncertainties that abounded, and the potential consequences of misjudging the seriousness of the tuberculosis epidemic, public health officials had little option other than to implement coercive health measures in support of their efforts to improve treatment completion rates and compliance. Economist John Maynard Keynes noted that, "as living and moving beings, we are forced to act . . . [even when] our existing knowledge does not provide a sufficient basis for a calculated mathematical expectation."[68] It was on this concept, rather than on objective evidence, that detention of noncompliant noninfectious individuals was based. While it is still unclear in late 1999 what impact the detention of noninfectious patients has had on the spread of the disease (no estimates have been made of the benefits gained), in terms of the number of cases prevented (excluding those who complied with treatment and were never detained) the number is likely to be small. The impact the threat of detention had on compliance and thereby on the development of drug resistance is a separate question (which was addressed earlier, in chapter 2).

The anxiety over multidrug-resistant tuberculosis in New York has now largely abated. It will be interesting to see if, in response, either the regulations or the application of them is modified. The real test is whether, in a decade or so, these measures are still in use, and, if they are, whether they are based on an explicit analysis of public health benefit or on the same subjective beliefs. With the widespread promotion of directly observed therapy, especially by the World Health Organization, will it be necessary to underpin these programs in other affluent nations with coercive measures? And will the public health measures advanced be culturally sensitive and not simply based on perceived successes elsewhere where the circumstances and the goals were different? Inap-

propriate, ill-judged, culturally insensitive coercive public health measures may hinder more than help global control of tuberculosis.

The future freedom of those individuals with tuberculosis who
refuse to comply with treatment is uncertain. It is ironic that this failure
to conform was questioned first in the land of freedom, liberty, and
multicultural tolerance.

Culture, Morality, and Tuberculosis

Give me your tired, your poor,
Your huddled masses yearning to breathe free . . .

—Emma Lazarus, *The New Colossus,* 1883

Why did the tuberculosis epidemic occur in New York City? Why was coercion thought to be a necessary part of the public health armamentarium to respond to the threat of widespread multidrug-resistant tuberculosis in the United States? The answers to these questions are complex but in many ways highlight the tensions present in most Western industrial societies (and, indeed, many of the emergent postcommunist Eastern bloc regimes). Of fundamental importance is the changing tension between individual responsibilities and societal duties and obligations. If tuberculosis highlights not only public health failures but also societal weaknesses (in failing to provide succor to the marginalized and vulnerable), then, if the notion that coercion was an effective control tool is accepted, the need for coercion to control tuberculosis also highlights a failure of many individuals' obligations to society. The New York City tuberculosis epidemic threw into stark relief, at least to this visitor, some of the fundamental societal and cultural questions currently being asked in the United States and Europe. To what extent should society protect and offer assistance to the needy? To what extent should market forces be constrained in the broader interests of society, and in particular in the interests of those less able to "compete"? How can the tensions between unabated individualism and communal responsibility be resolved? What is the role of government in effecting societal change? (Many, at least in the United States, would say that government cannot [indeed some would say *should* not] even attempt to mold society. The contempt with which the notion of social engineering is regarded in the United States provides a sense of this.) To what extent has the deep cynicism of the people toward politics and politicians affected the politicians' role?

Looking at public health failures and successes only through the narrow biomedical lens fails to reveal many, and perhaps the most important, lessons available. For a more complete understanding of tuberculosis, we require more than simply understanding who is at risk and applying efforts to track, diagnose, and treat them. How cultural, societal, and political forces conspire to influence the development of an epidemic such as that seen in New York and determine the response must be considered. Unless this is done policies that may have been successful under one set of conditions, in one society, in one country, may be transferred to other settings although they are unsuccessful or inappropriate in the new situation.

This chapter examines some of the sociological, political, and cultural tensions that both provoked the epidemic and dictated the response to it. These tensions are present in all Western nations to some degree, yet in the United States, and most especially in New York City, they are more tangible than elsewhere, the forces more powerful. While these tensions also exist in Europe, their quality is different. As a consequence, the tone of debate regarding the most vulnerable is also different. This chapter addresses the culture of individuality, explores the idea of community and issues surrounding social cohesion, examines the influence of morality and how American ideas on morality have influenced policy, and touches on how politics and political ideology are determining responses.

EXCEPTIONALISM

Declining social capital and increasing social exclusion particularly affect the poorest members in a society. In those already marginalized and vulnerable the development of a communicable disease such as tuberculosis provokes little sympathy from others, and from the individual affected it may promote hostility and further isolation.

In 1997 the *New York Times* ran a special magazine issue entitled "New York's Parallel Lives." In the main article the author discounts earlier metaphors for the diversity of the city (a melting pot, a boiling pot, a rainbow, a patchwork quilt, a gorgeous mosaic) and uses the image of the Central Park "Skate Circle" instead. The circle consists of a group of roller skaters, who have congregated in the park for twenty years or so and who all tune their radios to the same station and dance together.

> At first glance the Skate Circle seems to be one great melting pot, one big happy family of man. But of course it's not quite that simple, or friendly. Most of the skaters barely know one another. They arrive separately and leave separately, and as they perform for the international crowd of spectators, they're concentrating on their moves, not on their brother and sister skaters. These dancers, skating side by side, crammed together competing for attention, are a model of the city's chaotic social structure, an assortment of subcultures that occasionally overlap but are mostly oblivious to one another.[1]

The article, which captures some of the vibrancy and diversity of the city, also suggests that the social forces between disparate groups is weaker than many would hope. Furthermore, although the Skate Circle may illustrate New York City's social networks, it also sheds light on "communities" throughout the nation and supports recent research findings that suggest that America's social fabric is increasingly stressed. There is little communication between groups, groups are segregated, and, by extension, the support groups give each other is stressed. Each group, or individual, increasingly views each other group as "different," emphasizing a "them" and an "us." Social cohesion is weak and social engagement is increasingly shallow.

Why is this so? Chapter 3 described how social networks in poor neighborhoods were destroyed in the 1970s and 1980s due to a combination of neglect and willful disregard. But the stress on the social fabric affects not one or even several small poverty-stricken areas; rather it involves whole cities. Certainly the heterogeneity of the New York City contributes to this failure to "mix," because of cultural and language differences. In addition, class differences and the wide extremes of wealth explain some of this intergroup ignorance. Beyond even these barriers, however, there is still a lack of integration and trust. Certainly individuals of different races, cultures, and backgrounds mix at work. But socially they frequently do not, particularly the most poor. Racial segregation is a remarkable feature of America. The black militancy of earlier decades may have encouraged this, but even now interracial relationships are infrequent. Alexis de Tocqueville, the French commentator on U.S. social mores, noted this divide between blacks and whites 150 years ago when he observed: "The two races are bound one to the other without mingling; it is equally difficult for them to separate completely or to unite. . . . You can make the Negro free, but you cannot prevent him facing the European as a stranger."[2] In the 1960s Senator Daniel Patrick Moynihan, referring to black poverty and alienation, what he termed a "tangle of pathology," commented: "The present generation of Negro youth growing up in the urban ghettos has probably less personal contact with the white world than any generation in the history of the Negro American."[3] New York City is one of the most segregated cities in America—along with Chicago, Detroit, Cleveland, and Milwaukee. In the 1980s, regardless of their incomes, blacks and whites remained as segregated as ever. Most blacks live in residential blocks or groups of blocks in which 75 percent or more of the population is also black; the picture is little different for Hispanic segregation. In the United States race segregates more than income. Yet this segregation has not produced separate cohesive minority groupings. Large sections of most minorities have gained economic and societal benefits, leaving behind socially excluded, ghettoized poor subpopulations. The result of this economic "bifurcation" described by Harvard sociologist William Julius Wilson and Princeton political economist Richard Nathan has resulted in a geographical separation and further disturbed communities.[4] How much of the racial separation is through choice rather than necessity is difficult to gauge, but the effect is much the same: a loss of sympathetic understanding between and within groups. Choice certainly seems important. Personal ads in New York magazines almost invariably seek same-race contacts (of whatever sexual orientation). In 1970 census data showed that under 1 percent of all marriages were interracial. In 1990 the rate was still under 2 percent. In New York, where approximately 50 percent of the population is nonwhite, mixed couples (other than white-Asian) are a rare sighting, and black-white couples especially so. There is little more social intermingling of the races than there was in de Tocqueville's time, and much of the interracial contact is strained.[5] But even given the lack of racial mixing plus deepening inequality, loss of opportunity for some, changes in expectations, and community breakdown, social fragmentation appears to have increased in recent years and social networks across America have declined.

In 1995 Robert Putnam, the Harvard sociologist, drew attention to this decline in social networks and with it the deterioration of civil society in America in his widely read essay, "Bowling Alone: America's Declining Social Capital."[6] He defined "social capital" as the "features of social organization such as networks, norms, and social trust that facilitate coordination and cooperation for mutual benefit." In his article describing a decline in social capital, he outlined a reduction in civic engagement over the past 25 years, from voter turnout (down to less than 50 percent in the 1996 presidential election, the lowest on record), involvement in public meetings, engagement in civic organizations and associations, to bowling in organized leagues. In each area he described a reduction in involvement. Social capital was declining, he concluded, and with it organized forces such as trust. One of the few areas of communal behavior he documented that had not declined significantly was religious affiliation. This was the exception and highlighted rather than contradicted his thesis. Religion in America, he observed, was often not bound to institutions but is more "self-defined" or individualistic. A version, albeit probably exaggerated, of this individualistic approach was recently provided by a 26-year-old disabilities counselor who described herself as a "Methodist Taoist Native American Quaker Russian Orthodox Buddhist Jew."[7] It is somewhat difficult to imagine that her religious conviction(s) bind her to many others. Presumably she is somewhat isolated in her religious convictions. The overall picture is one of increasing social isolation and mistrust. Putnam suggests a number of reasons for this erosion of social capital; these include the changing role of women in the workforce (leaving both the house and the neighborhood to work), increased residential mobility, technology (particularly television),[8] personal computers, changing family makeup, and other demographic transformations that he alludes to but does not document. These would include, presumably, particularly with regard to the poor, many of the social changes detailed in chapter 2 that isolate and marginalize large sections of poor urban populations.

Putnam is not alone in documenting this changing social landscape. In 1996 the *Washington Post* ran a series of front-page articles highlighting research findings of a national survey that it conducted with Harvard University and the Kaiser Family Foundation. The overall findings in the first article, entitled "Americans Losing Trust in Each Other and Institutions" were summed up in this way: "America is becoming a nation of suspicious strangers, and this mistrust of each other is a major reason Americans have lost confidence in the federal government and virtually every other major national institution. Every generation that has come of age since the 1950s has been more mistrusting of human nature, a transformation in the national outlook that has deeply corroded the nation's social and political life." For example, in response to the question "Would you say that most people can be trusted or that you can't be too careful in dealing with people?" only 35 percent answered that most people can be trusted.[9] In a similar survey conducted in 1964, 54 percent had given this answer.[10]

In addition to temporal changes in the level of distrust and social cohesion, cross-sectional variations could be seen in the 1980s. As one would expect, the levels of distrust were not uniform across the country. Those states with marked inequality, for example, New York and many southern states, showed the highest levels of mistrust. Indeed, the correlation between inequality and mistrust was high.[11] On this basis one might have expected the same level of mistrust to have been amplified in major cities, such as New York City, Los Angeles, and Miami. It is therefore perhaps no coincidence that the cities with substantial numbers of "recalcitrant" tuberculosis patients were those displaying marked inequality. In New York, with its great disparities of income and wealth, desperate urban poverty neighboring ostentatious affluence, communities and individuals became, in the 1980s, more and more insular. With the scourge of drugs, poor economic opportunities, and the corresponding rise in crime, fear exacerbated this sense of isolation and distrust.

Other factors might have influenced the decline in social capital and may be useful to explore to further understand the causes and response to the tuberculosis epidemic. One is the cult of individualism, which historically has been profoundly influential in shaping the American cultural arena.

INDIVIDUALISM AND AUTONOMY

Individualism and autonomy have long been cornerstones of the American psyche. De Tocqueville remarked upon this self-reliance, this rugged individualism, autonomy, and independence of spirit, this "frontier mentality," in the nineteenth century. "The inhabitant of the United States learns from birth that he must rely on himself to combat the ills and trials of life; he is restless and defiant in his outlook toward the authority of society and appeals to its power only when he cannot do without it."[12] More than 30 years ago social commentator Seymour Martin Lipset, in his discourse on American values, emphasized two themes, individualism and equality, both of which, he believed, defined Americans and set them as a nation apart from others—American exceptionalism.[13] Regarding his country 30 years later, he continues to see the emphasis on individualism as a key characteristic differentiating the United States from other countries.[14] But this reverence for individuality is strained when individuals' deviant behavior threatens, or is perceived to threaten, the public health.

This accent on individualism can be seen more readily in the United States than elsewhere both because of the country's greater affluence and also because of the influence of history. Free will—the freedom to own property and to worship, speak, travel, promote one's self-interest, pursue happiness, have choice—has been integral to the American ethos since the days it was an agrarian society. The nation was founded on these ideals. Increasing cultural complexity and societal heterogeneity has further strengthened the forces of individualism. In a pluralistic multicultural society individuals' personal values naturally differ widely. But the forces enhancing individualism strain community bonds. Furthermore, in the late twentieth century the impact of science and technology, the mass media, television in particular, and the bureaucratic nature of modern society mean that Americans believe their possibilities and choices have expanded. At the same time cultural diversity has weakened community cohesion, and with these changes the accepted norms of behavior have become broader. Some constants persist, however, such as belief in American exceptionalism: America is the land of opportunity, individualism, and individual freedom.

Sociologist Ralf Dahrendorf has suggested that many of the more recent shifts seen in Western culture (e.g., from collectivism to individualism) have occurred to balance choices and bonds.[15] Choices enhance individualism and autonomy while bonds encourage social cohesion and stability. Individualism and personal freedom are constrained in societies where the bonds linking people are tight, but when individuals broaden their sphere of influence and of choice, the bonds are weakened. Over the past 50 years individuals have become less reliant on one another and have sought greater choice, but at the expense of weakening the social ties that bound them to their communities. And with these weakening ties the sense of social obligation has been weakened and the definition of social norms extended. This trend, it has been suggested, has resulted in the United States becoming an "over-optioned" society.[16]

Three powerful forces—ideology, affluence, and cultural heterogeneity—have conspired to make America the individualistic capital of the world. And New York City, the cultural and media capital of America— the Mecca of those most eccentric—is surely the individualistic capital of America.

Many commentators have described the uneasy balance between collectivism and individualism. A society that moves too far in one direction is likely to be unstable. Excessive collectivism results in tyranny and suppression of individual rights and initiative as seen, for example, in the former Soviet Union or in Mao Zedong's China. But a society that has moved too far in the other direction, toward unfettered individualism, may witness problems arising from alienation of those excluded from the social order through a lack of talent, skills, or opportunity. Some political commentators have talked in terms of pendulum swings between collectivism and individualism. Once one has experienced the freedom to express one's individuality, it may be difficult to return to a more constrained environment. The pendulum swings will not be smooth. And whether the pendulum will swing back in the foreseeable future which seems unlikely (given increasing globalization and global political trends) or whether it will continue wavering at one end of its arc is a legitimate question. If social harmony is dependent on a balance between individualism and collectivism, on the fulfillment of individual desires and collective needs, individual rights and civil responsibilities, then urban American (and indeed Western) society appears unbalanced at the moment. Although there is real academic and political enthusiasm for developing a more collectivist approach to resolving social ills, how this can be achieved and what form it will take is very uncertain.

In part, some of the tension between collectivism and individualism may relate to a popular misunderstanding of what individualism means.[17] To many it is a moral ideal, describing a personal search for self-fulfillment, or, in philosopher Charles Taylor's diction, "authenticity."[18] But another meaning, and one that has become widely, if erroneously, accepted, is that individualism is an amoral phenomenon. Individualism here means egoism, self-centeredness, the narrow pursuit of happiness with little regard for others or one's responsibilities to society. The rise of this second type of individualism, or social atomism, brings with it chaos and anomie. This "radical" or "expressive" individualism is devoted to self-aggrandizement. Such individualists are narcissistic and self-oriented and show little regard for groups or the public good (unless it directly affects their well-being). Libertarian economist Freidrich Hayek, among others, noted this divergence in the understanding of individualism, between individual responsibility and freedom on one hand, and mere egoism on the other when he wrote, "the belief in individual responsibility . . . has always been strong when people firmly believed in individual freedom" and later observed, with regard to self-serving individuality, that individual responsibility "has markedly declined, together with esteem for freedom."[19] De Tocqueville, too, noted the differences and predicted their merger in America:

> "Individualism" is a word recently coined to express a new idea. Our fathers only knew about egoism.
>
> Egoism is a passionate and exaggerated love of self which leads a man to think of all things in terms of himself and to prefer himself to all.
>
> Individualism is a calm and considered feeling which disposes each citizen to isolate himself from the mass of his fellows and withdraw into the circle of family and friends; with this little society formed to his taste, he gladly leaves the greater society to look after itself.
>
> Egoism springs from a blind instinct; individualism is based on misguided judgment rather than depraved feeling. It is due more to inadequate understanding than to perversity of heart.

> Egoism sterilises the seeds of every virtue; individualism at first only dams the spring of public virtues, but in the long run it attacks and destroys all others too and finally merges in egoism.[20]

The "recalcitrant" individual with tuberculosis is perhaps, therefore, simply exhibiting a behavioral trait at the end of a spectrum that is revered in the West, that of individualism. This is not surprising. Conflicting messages are sent from a society that encourages diversity of opinion and behavior, a skepticism of authority, individuality (both moral and amoral) and the rejection of conformity, compliance and deference while at the same time the social networks, the implicit social forces, which constrain destructive aberrant behavior are broken by society. Is it any wonder that "recalcitrance" is so much more obvious in the United States and, in particular, New York City? This extreme social atomism is well illustrated by the comments of one patient detained in Roosevelt Island's Goldwater Memorial Hospital. In referring to the reasons for her chaotic and antisocial behavior, she remarked: "I was seeking happiness by any means possible, it didn't matter how. It didn't matter if I hurt somebody, nobody could stop me getting happy." Later she commented, "I wanted to be 'down,' be in the in crowd. Wanted to be part of the gangsters—they was [sic] exciting. My life was so boring. They appeared to be doing all right, money in their pocket, cars, smoking reefer."

But this emphasis on individualism also determines, more broadly, in subliminal ways, social policy. Americans tend to individualize success, failure, and inequality, viewing them as resulting from individual differences, talents, and will rather than *circumstances*. If someone is successful it is because of who they intrinsically are or what they did.[21] The advantages society laid before them were inconsequential. This belief means that institutionalized social inequities (in contrast to violated individual rights) are harder to remedy. But institutionalized social advantages *do* exist and *do* matter. Children from impoverished backgrounds *do* benefit from improved educational resources, college education does improve earning potential, increased family support does reduce family breakdown, and good access to healthcare does improve health.[22] This individualization of policy also has consequences for those at the bottom of the heap. Just as those who "succeeded," by whatever measure one uses, did it on their own, those who "failed" also did it on their own. They failed because they did not try hard enough or were unlucky enough to be born with insufficient talent. Opportunities were open to them, they just did not grasp them. Circumstances were unimportant. Inequity does not exist.

This increasing American communal insularity and division into ever smaller groups was recently highlighted in another *New York Times Magazine* article.[23] Vermont is a state that has prided itself on its sense of being a special community. Most residents regard themselves as "liberal," many are affluent, and they are predominantly white. But an illuminating division has arisen between two neighboring towns over the public education of the towns' children. One town spends considerably more on each child's education than the other. The children going to the prosperous school, not surprisingly, benefit. But the State Supreme Court, in 1997, ruled this system unconstitutional; consequently legislators have started taking funds from prosperous "gold" towns to give to "receiver" towns via a change in property taxes. Vermonters are at each other's throats over this redistribution. "This is Marxism, not democracy," commented author and Vermonter John Irving. But this breakdown in community spirit represents more than an argument over redistribution. "The divisions that exist in all societies—between rich and poor, employer and employee, young and old, insiders and outsiders—are widening into chasms." Vermonters in neighboring towns do not now see each other as being from the same community, of the "same tribe," to use Columbia physician Karen Brudney's evocative phrase, they see a "them" and an "us." Quite how urban New York City public school children would view the squabble is unclear. What is clear, however, is that they receive considerably fewer benefits and educational resources and support than their affluent "neighbors." If redistribution between Vermont and New York was advocated, think of the uproar that would ensue. But inequities in school finances, which are largely locally determined, leave less-advantaged children way behind in the competition that ensues after they have left school.

In recent years there has been a shift away from Washington-directed social policy towards local and state-determined program in a range of issues, from environmental protection and crime, to sexual morality and welfare. This, as one commentator has noted, "raises deep questions about the virtues of direct democracy, the merits of federalism and the possibility of isolating states from national society."[24] Centralized strategic thinking is tied to "Big Government" and is currently largely unsupported.

What are the consequences of this fracturing of communities and emphasis on individualism? It means that individuals withdraw from each other and that society is increasingly split into ever smaller groups, each fearful of the others. It means the breakdown of a sense of common values, goals, trust, and sympathy for others' problems.

REDISTRIBUTION, JUSTICE, AND HEALTHCARE

This individual and group separateness and self-reliance is reflected in the attitude of Americans to redistribution of wealth, antagonism toward universal programs, enthusiasm for means-testing, and voluntarism. Moreover, this emphasis on self-reliance, individual responsibility, and decline in community spirit has meant that welfare support programs continue to divide the "deserving" from the "undeserving." In political parlance, programs now demand "reciprocity"; that is, people should "no longer expect something for nothing." Reciprocity, or mutuality, is defining future social policies rather than need-based entitlements.[25] This situation can be seen most clearly in the recent welfare reform. Similar changes in policy emphasis, in an attempt to stave off welfare dependency, are happening elsewhere—in the United Kingdom, for example.[26] This policy shift in both countries emphasizes individual obligations, not societal obligations. Inequities in education and social infrastructure responsible for failing to broaden equal opportunity receive little attention—which is somewhat surprising.

Americans passionately believe in equality, particularly when it comes to raising children or to political rights. Indeed, a society grounded in a commitment to equality of opportunity, a meritocracy, in addition to the possibility of a better life for each succeeding generation, is what defined writer James Truslow Adams's "American Dream."[27] Equality of opportunity is one of the cornerstones of the American national personality. Over 95 percent of Americans agree that "everyone in America should have equal opportunities to get ahead."[28] But, as political scientist Jennifer Hochschild and others have shown, in a land dedicated to equality of opportunity, there is a sizable gap between rhetoric and reality.[29] Americans accept enormous inequality in outcome, largely through choice, but they also accept widespread inequality of opportunity or inequity, largely unknowingly. I mentioned some of the institutionalized inequities present in society such as widespread child poverty, earlier. These problems have not been remedied, and there is little evidence that they will be. In fact, they hardly register in the concerns of most people. Yet if one believes that equality of opportunity or life-chance is a central tenet of a just society, as most Americans do, then one should at least consider why these inequities persist and attempt to redress them. Some projects, such as Head Start, have had some success in addressing problems early in an attempt to "level the playing field," but most receive little attention and support. As Daniel McMurrer and Isabel Sawhill, authors of *Getting Ahead*, recently commented, "[E]ven where such efforts have been effective, they have been grossly inadequate to the task of compensating for differences in early environment. The result is that the distribution of income is not just unequal. It is, to a greater extent than our public rhetoric would suggest, predictable."[30] A U.S. Assistant Attorney General noted recently, for example, "Society's collective thinking on the meaning of opportunity seems to begin and end with the topic of affirmative action," emphasizing the nation's preoccupation with race, to the detriment of addressing other institutionalized inequities and poverty.[31]

President John F. Kennedy, in 1963, questioned why the poor did not demand change, why they were not "angrier and more politically demanding."[32] The answer is multifactorial. In part it is because they are not a cohesive group; they do not speak with one voice; they are fragmented into different economic classes, religions, races, regions, and cultures; and they see, not the commonalties that bind them but the differences that separate them. Individuality plays a part both in the belief in the "American Dream" and a deeply held belief in self-reliance.

One of the most renowned North American thinkers on justice in recent decades is John Rawls. In his *A Theory of Justice*, Rawls challenged efficiency-based utilitarianism and proposed a principle of social justice that he described as "justice as fairness."[33] He promoted the idea that a just society must "genuinely" provide equality of opportunity. But he also suggested, contrary to libertarian equality ideals, that in order "[t]o treat all persons equally, to provide genuine equality of opportunity, society must give more attention to those with fewer native assets and to those born into less favorable social positions." Obviously, Rawls's theory of justice has not been practically applied. A theory of justice committed to equalizing opportunity should, one could argue, offer good healthcare and education to all. These areas are deserving of special attention since both are inextricably tied to equality of opportunity. One cannot take advantage of opportunities if one is ill or ill-educated. Adequate provision of both determines access to later goods and opportunities in life.[34] Yet, in the United States healthcare is a privilege, and, it could be argued, so, too, is a good education. Arguments that expansion of these services is "too expensive" are disingenuous. The choice to restrict public services, an explicit choice made by government with the implicit support of the populace and explicit support of powerful lobbyists, is made to *appear* unavoidable. As lawyers Guido Calabresi and Philip Bobbit point out in their book *Tragic Choices,* "By making the result [of a tragic choice] seem necessary, unavoidable, rather than chosen, [policymakers] attempt to convert what is tragically chosen into what is merely a fatal misfortune."[35] A charade is promoted which suggests that, for example with healthcare, all who need care can get it (through emergency departments). Yet with healthcare there is a real choice between restricted access with reduced costs and equal access with increased costs. The choice produces a conflict in values, between promoting equality of opportunity (through universal health coverage) and providing good care only for those who are able to afford it. Political institutions and powerful lobbyists in some ways deny this tragic choice so that society can avoid addressing "the costs of fundamental values in conflict." Society avoids having to make morally difficult decisions, for, once the choice is recognized for what it is, then "failure to choose is dishonest."[36] An alternative view is that U.S. society is clear about the choices: Inequity and limited redistribution of resources or equity and redistribution. It has chosen the first. The price of improving equality of opportunity through universal health provision is not worth paying because, first, it demands a more profound acceptance of redistribution such that some will pay for others' care, and second, it implies that some who are "undeserving" of coverage benefit.

Choosing between inequity and equity is so difficult because expanding healthcare access and coverage and improving education would entail greater redistribution of wealth than occurs currently. Americans largely support moves (although they rarely occur) to expand opportunity but reject moves toward equalizing outcome (even if they themselves would benefit). Redistribution receives little support. Complementing this attitude, Americans are nothing if not reluctant to pay more taxes. Americans hate paying taxes, much more so than Europeans, who simply grumble. Remember, President Bush failed to get reelected because he reneged on his promise, "Read my lips—no new taxes." This reluctance to pay taxes results, in part, from skepticism (often well founded) regarding the promise that taxes will be spent efficiently and wisely but also results from a peculiarly American attitude to redistribution of wealth. Although Americans believe in equality, they also believe in economic differentials and a rough, individualistic economic justice. This contrasts with the European attitude. During the Thatcher "revolution," a British Social Attitudes survey showed that most people favored paying more taxes if the least well off would benefit. This fact is somewhat paradoxical when one considers that the British, unlike most other Europeans, also perceive that the poor are lazy and lack willpower, which is similar to many American's attitude.[37] In contrast, a recent poll for Fox TV found American opinion divided two to one against a similar proposition regarding redistribution through taxation.[38] In another (international) survey, only about a quarter of Americans agreed that government should reduce income differences.[39]

Increasing inequality obviously serves to distance the common experiences between those at either end of the spectrum and reduce the cohesive bonds that allow society to function as a whole. Failure of opportunity gives rise to the tunnel effect discussed earlier and leads to greater hostility within society. This increase in social exclusion (i.e., the loss of access to the most important life chances, the ones that connect individuals to the mainstream of life) is felt most acutely by the poor, but by no means exclusively. The poor have fewer resources from which to draw, which exacerbates their situation and makes their sense of exclusion more obvious and painful. But this isolation, this withdrawal from societal involvement, affects everyone. The costs of social exclusion, in welfare support, policing and the criminal justice system, and healthcare fall on the entire society, through the taxes paid for benefits and the costs of private insurance and protection. But more important, everyone's quality of life deteriorates as fear of others and anxiety over personal security increases. Ultimately we are all excluded from enjoying the full fruits of society, or, as Dostoevsky recognized, "We are all responsible for all."

CIVIL RIGHTS AND COMMUNITY FRAGMENTATION

How does society respond to these centrifugal forces separating individuals from each other, fracturing groups, and reducing community spirit? As in physics, equal and opposite forces play out; the law counterbalances separational forces.

The United States is, perhaps like all countries, a country of contradictions. Liberty, freedom, and tolerance are concepts more highly revered in America than almost anywhere else in the world. Yet in the United States one is more keenly aware of rules, regulations, and laws than anywhere else in the West. Forces encouraging diversity are counterbalanced by forces encouraging conformity. Yet, as I have described, those communal forces that once would have tempered aberrant behavior have been weakened, and the force of law has replaced them. And, as those communal forces become ever weaker, the force of calls for sterner and stiffer sanctions increase. The fear of lawlessness demands sterner discipline. In the United States minor infringements of laws frequently result in public humiliation and retribution on a scale not seen elsewhere. One is bombarded with rules and regulations, from multiple road signs dictating where and when one can park ("Don't even think about parking here"), to messages on beer bottles warning pregnant women not to drink, to long lists of what one can and cannot do on the subways. New York City's mayor, at the time of this writing, after having overseen the decline in the annual homicide rate from more than 2,000 to about 750 murders each year, is attempting to clamp down on jaywalkers, street vendors, taxi drivers, and those who play their music too loud. His sense of machismo is palpable. America incarcerates more of its own than any other Western nation. Coercion is a visible, tangible concept in American life. Things seem to be seen as black or white *[sic]*, and flexibility is not apparent. Coercion, be it compliance policy with DOT or detention for noncompliance with treatment, is acceptable in the United States where elsewhere it might culturally not be. And the force of law explicitly underpins this use of coercion.

In the United States the law assumes a cultural and political prominence not seen in other countries. This is principally because of its place at the heart of the Constitution and the Bill of Rights. This emphasis on rights, again, is uniquely American. The Bill of Rights—

the first 10 amendments made to the Constitution in 1789—defines the limits of government power and protects individuals from government excesses. This was its purpose. In order to protect liberty, the founding fathers erected legal and political structures and intentionally fragmented power in different institutions of government. They devised the Bill of Rights to protect the rights of individuals. This protection of powers flowed naturally from the built-in conflict between government and the governed. Today this conflict is represented by the sometimes overwhelming emphasis on the law. Not for nothing are there more than 900,000 lawyers in America.

But this emphasis on political and civil rights rather than societal obligations (or, put another way, societal and economic rights), despite having a long history, has developed the fervor seen today only over the last 40 years. During the Progressive era the accent was on paternal state intervention to cure societal ills. The belief that the state could be effective and should intervene for beneficial purpose in a wide array of social problems reached its peak during Roosevelt's New Deal era (late 1930s). Since then the belief that the state is ineffective when it intervenes has increased, and the question is less what should be done and more should anything be done. Historian David Rothman, in 1978, phrased this attitudinal shift well: "Convinced that paternalistic state intervention in the name of the common good has all too typically worked to their disadvantage, [the disaffected] are now determined to rid themselves of the onus of ostensibly protective and benevolent oversight and substitute instead a commitment to their own autonomy."[40] This cynicism regarding government intervention rose, not surprisingly, when cynicism in government institutions increased, with the Watergate scandal. According to Ira Glasser of the ACLU,

> The reimposition of the Bill of Rights upon the presidency during the 1973-74 impeachment campaign came precisely at the point when the movement to establish limits on the discretion of social institutions also reached its peak. The re-emergence of the original understanding politically came after a decade of effort to apply the original understanding socially. The Bill of Rights seemed finally to overcome the imperial presidency precisely when it was struggling to overcome the imperial school principal, the imperial caseworker, and the imperial state psychiatrist.[41]

Interestingly, belief in government, after a brief, albeit muted, renaissance in the early 1980s, is now at the same level as its nadir in the 1970s.[42] Scandals regarding lobbyists' power, campaign finance, "inappropriate" relationships in the White House, and deal-making continue to reduce public confidence in the institutions of the state.

According to David Rothman, emblematic of a cultural shift in the 1960s and 1970s from the unified vision of brotherhood proclaimed by Martin Luther King to a focus on individual autonomy and group interests (and with it the loss of any belief in the harmonizing potential of state intervention) was King's assassination and the rise to prominence of the Black Power movement, which gained strength after the civil rights leader's death.[43] The movement illustrated this move toward advancing social justice through conflict and isolation rather than via mutually shared interests within the community. The movement adopted a strategy of group differentiation that other groups subsequently emulated. With this loss of shared dreams and fracturing of interests within defined groups, from prisoners to the mentally ill, from homosexuals to the elderly, King's dream of unity slid ever farther into the background. Interest groups benefit from this strategy of conflict, but whether communities as a whole do is open to question. This emphasis on civil and political rights has led, I believe, to a neglect of societal responsibilities, a focusing on the trees and a failure to see the wood or forest. Conservatives in particular (although increasingly Democrats) call for greater individual responsibility but fail to recognize that the state can and should play a role in redressing the balance and making society more just. As he himself recognized, Adam Smith's free market "invisible hand" is just not dexterous enough to correct social injustices, particularly when, the cards are so heavily stacked against some individuals. Currently in the United States it seems that rights are respected but needs are neglected, individual duties are highlighted but societal obligations are ignored.

I do not intend to suggest that the Bill of Rights negates governmental power, but it does limit that power, or rather, the negative rights listed in the Bill are, in my opinion, insufficiently counterbalanced by positive rights. The Bill of Rights dictates what the state cannot do to its citizens—negative rights—but it also hampers the development positive rights, or "social rights," which define what the state owes its citizens. The Bill of Rights does not paralyze government's ability to meet social needs, but, through a subtle (and now not-so-subtle) encouragement toward group differentiation and individual autonomy, its application may enhance societal divisions and thereby augment government inertia. The vulnerable and disenfranchised are marginalized further, and support and assistance from government is not forthcoming. Those demands made by the poorest in society seem to reach either deaf ears or inert bodies.

POLITICS AND "THE NEEDS OF STRANGERS"

How does this fragmentation of society (in already heterogeneous "communities") and this emphasis on individualism play out for the weakest in society? And how is it that coercion is viewed as necessary when these factors come together most obviously, as in New York City? As I have briefly focused on, in developing policies from an individualistic slant, in fractured communities with weakening cohesive social bonds, it is perhaps simply a natural extension to view those on the margins as "different." The bonds of common sympathy become weaker, and emphasis shifts from a communal common purpose with shared responsibilities to the promotion of special interests and a change of perspective from "us" to "them and us." In rejecting the hypothesis, as many have, that society has little influence over behavior, and in accepting in principle St. Augustine's doctrine of original sin, that is, that some are "just born evil," one can start to absolve society of its duties and emphasize human failings as the result of inherent predetermined moral weaknesses. This moral thread runs through much of American social policy, both historically and currently.

Religion has been used in the past to prop up a fragile social order and as a force to bind communities. Indeed, the strength of the evangelical Christians over the past 20 years, and their presence in American policymaking, has been one of the most potent forces charging and changing American politics.

America is different from other Western industrial nations. Its citizens are more religious and pious, racial divisions arouse deeper emotions, criminal violence and the "gun culture" is more prevalent, and the control of intoxicants, from alcohol, through illicit drugs, to smoking, has been more distressing for the American people (and its politicians) than for citizens in any other country. In an analysis of the differences between the American and European psyche, a recent commentator remarked: "The interconnections of Puritanism, racial conflict, criminal violence, the proliferation of firearms, the mania for incarceration and the prohibition of intoxicants are tight and unmistakable. Pull any of these threads and the rest are drawn along."[44] Or as Gore Vidal, that unmistakable observer of American culture, said in 1975 in his typically caustic fashion, there is a "deeply American delight in the punishing of others."[45] Moral images and moral stereotypes swim through the American cultural landscape. Personal morality is important in America and dictates policy to a greater extent than in any other industrial nation.

This was clearly seen when, in the 1980s, President Reagan responded to the desire of the American people for a new authority and national direction by promising a return to an America "strong at home and strong abroad." A rebirth in the attention paid to personal morality ensued. Social ills arose from not social injustice but laziness, greed, and lack of discipline. The "undeserving," the "unworthy" would not be carried any more on the backs of hardworking Americans. Only the truly needy or "those who through no fault of their own must depend on the rest of us" could rely on support. Those "with true need can rest assured that the social safety net of programs they depend on are exempt from any cuts."[46]

In essence, this approach determines that individuals, not societal factors, are the cause of the problem. And, usefully, at least from a political standpoint, the "victims" are invariably of low socioeconomic status with little political influence. By focusing on the individual, the social conditions can largely be disregarded. The medicalization of aberrant behavior further distances social influence on disease from the disease itself and the individual sufferer. This means that the social forces that determine disease development to some degree (and the individual response to it) are left largely unrecognized and often unremedied.[47] So, for example, most of the articles published in the medical press during the New York City epidemic either ignored the social factors that undoubtedly had influenced the epidemic's expansion or merely skirted over the issue while suggesting the need for greater public health resources. The divorce between social policy and health seemed almost complete. Newspaper and magazine articles centered on the public health failures (and even this criticism was often muted) and the failures of individuals to comply with treatment. Broad social inequities were hardly touched on.

The ongoing popular public discussion on public policy has put many broad social and economic ills squarely on the shoulders of individuals. Welfare dependency, poor performance in school, unemployment, criminal behavior, and even some types of illhealth (e.g., HIV and other sexually transmitted diseases) often are seen simply as the result of personal shortcomings. The individualization of social problems squares well with the emphasis on individualism. It means that the focus regarding the causes and solutions to social problems is thrust on the individual alone rather than the society. It exonerates society, and any institutionalized inequities are merely aberrations of little significance. This abdication of societal obligations encourages the "victim" to be blamed for society's ills, and fits well with American Calvinistic values.[48] The breakdown of community spirit amplifies the presence of "strangers," that invidious social group. And the "needs of strangers" will not be provided for.[49]

The estrangement of the poor from the mainstream of society had become acceptable (again) with Reagan's ideological shift and had been practically augmented by his policies. "Morality" had an insidious effect. Federal support for a broad range of social safety nets declined, in part because of an ideological attack on government intervention in social policy but also as an attack on "undeserving" individuals who were taking advantage of "generous" welfare support to avoid work. Overcrowding, increased inequality and poverty, and the fracturing of neighborhoods were some of the more obvious consequences.

Current policies aimed at alleviating poverty continue to have moral undertones, sometimes ironic ones. For example, Clinton's welfare reform (under the gloriously named 1996 Personal Responsibility and Work Opportunity Act) may be effective in reducing welfare rolls and even encourage those intent on work to seek it. But it contains a moral element that has not been widely debated. Much of the moral rhetoric regarding the "welfare dependent" has been aimed at single mothers (implicitly black and never married, rather than white and divorced). The family values advocated by many conservatives advance the notion that "a mother's place is in the home" with her children, despite the fact that most women with children work. These values, presumably, therefore, hold only for middle-class mothers. Poor single mothers should be out working (which, presumably, makes them irresponsible mothers at the same time because they are leaving their children in somebody else's care). Ironically, many mothers are leaving the welfare rolls to become poorly paid child care workers looking after other mothers' children.[50] A further example where morality weighs heavily on welfare recipients, has occurred in the screening for drug and alcohol addiction. In future, benefits will be halted for those who refuse to be screened, and obviously the consequences will be felt by both the adults and their children.[51]

The moral overtones castigating those on welfare obscure a paradox. Americans care deeply about the poor. As a nation, they give more money per capita in voluntary contributions than any other nation on earth. For example, in 1991 Americans gave $125 billion to private charities, many of them religious organizations, which feed the homeless, clothe poor children, and so on.[52] Yet they have little sympathy for those on welfare. Despite evidence to the contrary, there is a deeply held belief that welfare discourages individuals from working, breaks up two-parent families, and encourages unmarried women to bear children.[53] Dependency breeds contempt among most Americans. Yet need is recognized for what it is. If, despite hard work and moral rectitude, one is still in need of support, then this is one's due. But if one cannot effectively project these character traits, then one is assumed to be work-shy, have poor moral fiber, and be undeserving of sympathy and support.

This enthusiasm to "blame the victim" can be seen beyond the broad arena of poverty. Just as poverty and welfare dependency are blamed on character flaws, so too are drug abuse, homosexuality, sex outside marriage, HIV, and homelessness. Greater virtue, it has been argued, would remedy all of these problems.[54]

HIV par excellence highlights the moral failings of many. In 1995 Senator Jesse Helms, in arguing that funding for AIDS programs should be reduced, summed up his and many other conservatives' views on those infected with HIV when he suggested that those with the disease had contracted it through their own "deliberate, disgusting, revolting conduct." His ire was obviously focused on homosexuals and drug users. But, as sociologist Erich Goode suggested when quoting him, his moral outrage was presumably not focused on hemophiliacs, those who had received contaminated blood products, children of infected mothers, or others who had acquired the infection "through no fault of their own."[55] Helms was focusing "fault" on a disease. He believes that the virtuous do not get AIDS, and those with AIDS are undeserving of our sympathy and support. This stance is not new. In concert with the "nationwide crusade against drugs" and the passing of federal bills to enhance this effort in 1986, 1988, and 1992, the Reagan administration had, throughout the decade, opposed the expansion of HIV education programs, the development of needle exchanges, and had supported mandatory testing. Helms had been at the forefront of these conservative policies and even had advocated quarantine of those infected. These sentiments were not simply the rantings of an out-of-step far-right conservative.[56] It had taken years for President Reagan even to speak publicly of AIDS. Not until May 1987 did he finally give his long-awaited maiden statement on the epidemic, and he endorsed mandatory testing of specific groups (i.e., prisoners) and routine testing of applicants for marriage licenses.[57] The Reagan administration consistently thwarted the efforts of the Surgeon General, C. Everett Koop, from advancing realistic, pragmatic policies devoid of moralistic overtones. Abstinence was the answer: from sex outside marriage,[58] and abstinence from drugs. "Just Say No." One of the main protagonists of this "zero tolerance" policy was First Lady Nancy Reagan. In 1988 she told the press: "If you're a casual drug user, you are an accomplice to murder." More rabid, but extending the same line of thought, was the suggestion of Daryl Gates, then the Los Angeles police chief, that "casual drug users [should be] be taken out and shot."[59]

This reluctance to divorce public health from personal morality continues today. In New York City, with its substantial injecting drug user population, needle exchanges became officially acceptable only once it was clear pregnant women and their children were acquiring HIV. Thus the catalyst for the local development of needle exchange programs was heterosexual and perinatal transmission of HIV. Transmission between drug users resulting in large numbers of HIV-infected drug users was deemed acceptable, but "innocent" children with AIDS was not. At the federal level, this reluctance to endorse needle exchanges persists—there are still no federal programs. Needle exchanges both prevent HIV transmission and, crucially for the moralists, do not encourage drug use. It had been politically necessary to surmount this last hurdle before the federal ban on support could be lifted. Recent evidence has confirmed that needle exchanges did not encourage drug use. Despite this, and despite the fact that it has been estimated that with wider implementation of needle exchanges, infection would be prevented in approximately 12,000 individuals a year, *and* despite the support of most in his party and administration, in 1998 President Clinton reiterated his support for maintaining the federal ban instituted by Reagan.[60] As one commentator noted, in making this moral rather than practical decision, "Clinton showed he had lost none of his ability to agonize when forced to choose between the popular course and the right one." This approach has been mirrored across the country. In New Jersey, for example, a state with about 37,000 people with AIDS, half of whom acquired it through injecting drug use, the governor, Republican Christine Whitman, restated her opposition to needle exchange programs recently: "[They] represent a government blessing of illicit and dangerous drug use, plain and simple."[61] In another example, in Connecticut, a needle exchange program was abandoned recently after a two-year-old girl pricked her finger on a discarded needle she had found in her yard. The fact that children are acquiring HIV daily through vertical transmission at birth because their mothers have acquired the infection through needle sharing on a scale unseen elsewhere in the developed world seems altogether to escape "moralists." As of December 1997 more than 200,000 cases of AIDS reported to the Centers for Disease Control and Prevention were directly or indirectly associated with injecting-drug use.[62]

Although Clinton has eschewed the phrase "War on Drugs," he has held the populist baton firmly, and the "crusade" against drugs continues. The public health consequences, of which HIV spread and resurgent tuberculosis have been only two, have been of secondary importance to the short-term political benefits.

Cultural observer Seymour Martin Lipsett has written that Americans "tend to view social and political dramas as morality plays, as battles between God and the Devil, so that compromise is virtually unthinkable." This inability to compromise feeds notions of abstinence favored by moralists—from sexual abstinence for teenagers, sexual McCarthyism in the political arena, abstinence from alcohol for pregnant women, to bans on smoking in prisons because of the risks to others from passive smoking. The doctrine of absolute drug abstinence has produced, not surprisingly, many "collateral" casualties. Prison and jail populations are overflowing. More than 60 percent of federal prisoners are drug offenders, and almost 25 percent of state prisoners are. Local jails house an additional half-million people. Hordes of young men, mainly black, from the inner cities have been affected, with "poverty, alienation, and violent antisocial behavior" escalating and their communities being destroyed.[63] The cost of the "War on Drugs" has risen from $1 billion a year in 1975 to $16 billion a year today, most of it spent on enforcement. Nearly $300 billion has been spent so far in the war, yet cocaine and heroin are cheaper than ever and marijuana use in teenagers has doubled since 1990. Its use is widespread,[64] despite hefty penalties for marijuana use, the antidrugs campaigns, and the exhortations of politicians such as Senator Orrin Hatch (R-UT), the chairman of the Senate Judiciary Committee, who supports mandatory sentences and suggests that, with regard to marijuana users, "We ought to lock them up and throw away the keys."[65]

As with drug users, so too the "feckless" homeless have long been the focus of moral outrage. Through the 1980s and 1990s they continued to be stereotyped as beggars who were "malodorous and willfully annoying."[66] This occurred despite changes in the makeup of the homeless population, from largely single men and women, to young people, women with children, and families.[67] In the early 1990s the call went out not to increase housing availability but to increase screening to exclude from housing many who had been in the shelter system. "Lack of housing is not so much a problem for them as is an inability to function normally because of a variety of social problems—including drug or alcohol addiction, criminality and an inability or unwillingness to work," noted one journalist.[68] The number of those residing within the shelter system increased. The city did not have to offer more than shelter, as adequate housing is not a right. The responsibility of the homeless, it seems, was to remain out of sight.

AIDS, sex, prisons, homelessness, and drug policy are inextricably intertwined and have been fertile grounds for those bent on separating the virtuous from the flawed. And whereas public health officials responding to the tuberculosis epidemic in New York City were, by and large, eager not to feed the morally outraged, separating tuberculosis policy from wider social policies is all but impossible. Views on the moral turpitude of those most at risk of developing tuberculosis have undoubtedly influenced allied social policies, causing further marginalization and exclusion of those most in need of support. Indeed, some pragmatists have suggested that a practical merging of these policies would be to take advantage of high incarceration rates and target tuberculosis prevention strategies there. After all, "correctional institutions [are] the most frequent, and often only, potential public health site for tuberculosis prevention encountered" by many patients at risk of developing tuberculosis.[69]

CONCLUSION

A great paradox, it seems to me, underpins the use of coercion in the control of a contagious disease. A typical individual detained because of poor treatment compliance might be described as poor, black, HIV-infected, homeless, an ex-felon, who would likely have a drug problem.[70] In contemporary America, one would be hard put to describe any group of individuals less "deserving" of assistance. If tuberculosis was not contagious but simply caused ill health in the poor and underprivileged, undoubtedly such focused public health efforts would not have been mounted. The infectious nature of the disease demanded such an aggressive response, for it threatened to overspill the ghettos and affect the population at large. After all, the recognition of high mortality rates from other causes in ghettos had not resulted in such focused national public health efforts or expenditure

The paradox arises because Americans, as de Tocqueville noted 150 years ago, are singularly concerned with their own well-being. As a people they are extremely health conscious. Furthermore, they are highly sensitive to risks, particularly when those risks are novel or borne involuntarily. These features make health hazards such as HIV, tuberculosis, and other contagious diseases especially compelling for policymakers, the media, and the general public alike. This combination of health consciousness and "victim-blaming" usually causes few ripples because the two "ideologies" rarely cross. But public anxiety rises and demands a response with a contagious disease that affects "them," but can be transmitted to "us" "through no fault of our own." Ironically, this response requires great expenditure on those who are "undeserving." Therefore, the response is focused narrowly on those who may be the cause of contagion rather than on the causes of the conditions from which illness arose.

If long-term control of tuberculosis—elimination is, for the foreseeable future, impossible—is to be achieved, then a radical new approach is required. Not only do public health programs, which currently contain the disease, need to be guaranteed, but society needs to address its ills explicitly. Tuberculosis in New York City, in many ways, simply illustrates how an affluent society can still be plagued by a centuries-old curable and preventable contagion. The social fractures that encouraged its resurgence and hindered the response are still present—but hiding under millions of dollars spent on a narrowly focused public health program and an economic boom. Once the economic cycle takes a down-turn and resources for public health are cut, tuberculosis will resurface.

Respiratory physician Lee Reichman has drawn attention to how the incidence of tuberculosis changes with changes in program funding.[71] Yet tuberculosis is more complex than the result of underfunding of a tuberculosis program, and likewise the response to it demands a broader and more complex approach. Tuberculosis can be controlled by expending vast sums of money to patch up the holes in the social fabric, just as other public health threats can be remedied in this "Band-Aid" fashion. But the fundamental causal societal weaknesses persist; these need to be recognized so that we are not constantly patching up different parts of a slowly disintegrating garment. This is not public health nihilism but an attempt to argue that politics can and should play a role in the development of a socially more just, less divided society; this will benefit society itself, individuals currently most susceptible to coercive practices and exclusion, and the public health.

But Americans view the political institutions in the United States with deep skepticism. Ineffectual government, augmented by the unfettered power of lobbyists and organized special interest groups, reduces the influence of constituents. Narrow political interests hold sway over broad social problems. Even when there is popular support in principle for change, such as healthcare reform, powerful groups with substantial resources impede change. Voters neglect the polling booth in increasing numbers as their disenchantment with the political process grows. And at the heart institutional inertia created by the Constitution thwarts reform and reformers. James Morone, professor of political science at Brown University, addressed this when he said, "There comes a point where too many checks create their own mischief—inept administration, thin democracy, and the enmity of the people."[72] Too many checks blunt social change. Moreover, currently a political consensus overarches all social policy initiatives. And this overarching consensus is morally driven and therefore exclusive. Supermajorities in the House of Representatives have, in the past, implemented radical reform. But these have been on the back of collective adversity or when social problems were viewed as community problems, not as those of individuals. Today, social problems today are not seen through this lens; instead they are individual or narrowly defined group problems. Until they are seen as broad societal problems, little will change.

President Clinton recently called for a "national debate on race." The debate, I believe, should not be on race but on inequality of opportunity and the social role of government. Race is a substantial part, but only a part, of the debate. Indeed, race is often used as a proxy for the consequences of poverty. (Witness the current discussions on the rising HIV rates in blacks.) By concentrating on race, one risks emphasizing further differences, and group divisions become magnified. The argument in Vermont over education has resulted from emphasizing differences and a lack of shared communal goals. The failure to see that Americans in Vermont might have a goal in common with those in New York City, or in Chicago, where race as well as economics becomes part of the equation, illustrates how deep the divisions are. This "fixing of lines of division on ethnic and racial bases," this enthusiasm for "multiculturalism," has superseded earlier efforts toward assimilation under one American cultural umbrella.[73] Over the past 25 years the multicultural left has rejected the goal of an assimilated, integrated society. But over this same period the right, particularly the Christian fundamentalists, have vilified the federal government, incapacitating national strategic policies. These two opposing forces have had a similar effect: to further divide the nation and drive a wedge between common experiences and common goals.

Americans hold certain core values more closely to their hearts than citizens in other nations. One of these values is "fairness." The United States is a land dedicated to opportunity *for all*. All should have an equal chance from the starting blocks in life's race. Yet they do not. Inequity is widespread. Political rhetoric obscures this fact, and undue interest group influence on government obfuscates it. Perhaps now, with inequalities wider than they have been for 30 years, is the time to reflect on what Franklin Delano Roosevelt said in 1937: "[The] test of our progress is not whether we add more to the abundance of those who have much; it is whether we provide enough for those who have too little."[74] Tuberculosis is a social and political problem as much as it is a medical problem.[75] Only by addressing tuberculosis from all of these perspectives will the benefits of intervention be sustained.

Lessons for Europe

But things will be better, he tells us. Afterwards, to every question
he says simply, "Trust me."

—Gore Vidal reporting on Tony Blair, *Virgin Islands,* 1997

In the West, momentous events in the East, the dismantling of the Berlin Wall, the collapse of the Soviet Union and its communist system, have coincided with a time of increasing political homogeneity. As Donald Sassoon, the noted British historian, commented recently: "Irrespective of separate national traditions, economic particularities, contrasting social structures and cultural differences, the nations of the world are being enjoined to deregulate labor markets, to lower or eliminate tariffs, to privatize state property, to eliminate subsidies and, in general, to let market forces operate with as few impediments as possible."[1] Laissez-faire Thatcherite libertarianism has replaced both communism and Keynesian capitalism as the dominant political ideology of Europe, both East and West. Representative of this shift, the Labour Party, and now the Labour government in Britain, has repositioned itself as the center-left party, severing its ties with the trade unions and becoming pro business, rejecting collective ownership, and seeking, like the Clinton administration and others in Europe, a "Third Way."

Globalization of markets is one of the keys to this transformation. Isolated Keynesian policies within one nation are doomed to fail. The markets, highlighting unavoidable wider interdependence, are too powerful, a fact that was illuminated by the debacle in Europe of currency "shadowing" that led to Black Wednesday, Britain's withdrawal from the European exchange rate mechanism, and the stall in European monetary union in the early 1990s. Despite this, monetary union is a reality for the continent. It remains to be seen to what extent national politics will be constrained by the loss of local domestic control over the economy— and what the consequences of this loss of influence will be. But what is clear is the influence local politicians have over their national economic situation is less now than before.

Politics is further constrained by the media. The mass media, controlled by a dwindling number of individuals, determines the message, which, as its influence grows greater than that of the print media (which, again, is controlled by an ever smaller elite group), results in a simplified debate that revolves around sound bites. The media, rather than politicians, increasingly determine the direction and the boundaries of debate. Political messages are sloganized and homogeneous. Complex debate is stifled. More and more, the simple message emphasizes how policies will affect *you,* not the wider community, and politics has become more defensive and reactive, less proactive. Politicians increasingly follow public opinion rather than lead. The notions of unity and common purpose captured by the New Deal and, to a lesser degree, the Great Society in the United States, and Aneurin Bevan's Welfare State in Britain, are all becoming, or threaten to become, distant memories. The left's ill-defined new ideology, its "Third Way," lacks clarity in defining a view on the future of society, and the fear is that it is simply an attempt to shore up against the destruction of past achievements. Whether the markets will accept the modest aims of the "Third Way" is uncertain. The market is king. It determines which policies will be promoted. The left's rhetoric, which is in the ascendancy in the West after the right's domination of the 1980s and early 1990s, continues to speak of greater equality, greater opportunity, and greater social cohesion, but intervention to ensure this is, by political and economic necessity, limited. The market "lacks a social conscience."[2] As in the United States, societal responsibility increasingly, as a consequence, receives less attention and individual duties receive more. Increased civility is dependent on the encouragement of personal responsibility.[3]

In Britain Prime Minister Tony Blair has compared his political aims with those achieved after 1945 and has suggested that the national mood for change is analogous to that seen at the inception of the Welfare State.[4] However, Blair, like Clinton with his reminiscences of Roosevelt's New Deal, does not appear to have a coherent plan of social reform, is constrained by globalization and the markets (and in Clinton's case the institution of government and scandals), and there is little sense of national solidarity (which had occurred in earlier times through universal adversity): social cohesion and support is more friable. Radical pragmatic political shifts in ideology are not possible in the current climate or foreseeable future. Any change that occurs will be incremental. Politicians of the left across Europe are now far more limited in their scope to enhance social change. In this vein political scientist Colin Leys recently noted, regarding politicians, that "Achieving office and doing some good within the bounds set by 'global market forces' increasingly become the real limit of their aspirations."[5]

What is of particular concern is the increasing use of "morality" to determine worth and hence policies by European political parties. In Britain this was highlighted recently by journalist Tariq Ali, when he drew attention to the paucity of real ideas from the Labour Party for amending the Conservative's legacy of social deprivation: "Incapable of promoting policies to alleviate the suffering of the two million unemployed and millions of underprivileged citizens and thus help bring about a society more at ease with itself, our politicians instead have clambered onto the morality bandwagon."[6] Unfortunately, the Labour government's enthusiasm to retain the support of "middle England" support means it has adopted many of the values of "middle England."

In emerging postcommunist Eastern European countries, the ex-communist parties have remained the dominant parties of the left. (The Czech republic is an exception.) Many have changed their names to "social-democrat" or "socialist," but they remain ideologically committed to the left-wing. There has been a marked polarization between communism and anticommunism, which some have suggested has been encouraged by the West, and nationalism versus Europeanism. How these issues resolve themselves may profoundly affect the direction of future EU policy. If instability increases, and authoritarian populism gains greater support, control of communicable diseases will undoubtedly become more difficult, as history has repeatedly shown us. *M. tuberculosis* does not recognize borders, but it does seek chaos. Already venereal diseases are reaching epidemic proportions, HIV incidence is rising, and tuberculosis rates are increasing. What is of particular concern is that drug-resistant and multidrug-resistant tuberculosis is now common in some countries. Latvia, for example, has a prevalence of MDRTB of more than 14 percent; Estonia of 10 percent.[7] What impact poor control in some countries will have on others is unclear, but Finland and other Scandinavian countries bordering the Baltic States are concerned. How they will respond is unclear. Yet signs of rising nationalism, allied to economic woes, and anti-immigrant sentiments do not bode well. Coercive public health responses directed at immigrants and the poor regarding tuberculosis may well be seen in Western Europe as public anxiety rises in the years to come. Immigrants and refugees have historically been scapegoated when social insecurity rises. In Britain and elsewhere in the late 1990s, ire is increasingly being focused on immigrants, refugees, and those seeking asylum, and social support is being withdrawn by popular mandate. Poor housing, poverty, and malnutrition are part of daily life for many recent entrants, and with the recognized increased risks of tuberculosis, one can imagine how the fears surrounding the importation of disease will be fueled.[8]

Europe could learn much from the United States, which is, in effect, 50 countries weakly tied by a federal government with limited powers. Yet, despite this weak alliance, regional differences, and the geographical scale, the union holds together. Americans, given their diversity, broadly tolerate each other to a remarkable degree, and have done so for 200 years. This can hardly be said for Europe. In the twentieth century Europe has been plagued by two world wars, the second based on racial and ethnic hatred; the Balkan states are fractured by ethnic tensions; the "troubles" originating from religious intolerance in Northern Ireland persist. Despite the political homogeneity of the United States and Europe, the United States appears relatively culturally homogeneous, or at least culturally dissipated, with most of its citizens having a similar core set of values and aspirations. In Europe cultural heterogeneity persists and is regionally defined. Increasingly Europe is becoming less a continent of nation-states and more a continent of regions, each with its own cultural identity. This can be seen in several regions, from the dismantled Soviet Union and Eastern European states; through Germany with its powerful semiautonomous Länder; Spain's culturally, politically, and economically semi-independent Catalan region; to the recent devolution of power to Britain's Scotland and Wales. In the face of advancing globalization it is these protectionist cultural differences and the isolationist tendencies that threaten social harmony and thereby public health. An American commentator recently noted perceptively that Europe is not a group

> of self-contained, independent states, nor is it a cohesive European Union (EU). Power is shifting unevenly among capitals, Brussels-based institutions of the EU, and, most conspicuously, regional centers. The trends are fairly clear, Europe's capacity for seriously affecting them increasingly feeble. Little political or moral leadership is being exercised in most capitals. In London, Prime Minister Tony Blair's government does have energy and some direction, not to mention a strong mandate. Still, there is no agreement, let alone a shared vision, on how Europe in its various parts should be orga-nized.[9]

Tensions undoubtedly will increase as some regions become more prosperous and others are left behind. Those tensions will play out first upon society's weakest.

The differences between a federal Europe and the United States are vast, less political and economic than historical and cultural. In the United States the indigenous population was, in effect, removed, and most immigrants have entered in search of a better life, many escaping persecution in their home countries. Those who were not voluntary immigrants, the blacks, still bear the scars, and race, as a consequence, tests policymakers' minds perhaps more than any other issue. The country is new, and the divisions present have not had time to fester as they have in Europe. One need only look at Northern Ireland or the Balkan region to see how difficult it is to erase the hatred borne upon history. The diffuse diversity of the United States is its strength. No one group holds sway.

In Europe, with its relatively homogeneous populations concentrated in specific areas, some of which are gaining political authority, those who are "different" are more liable to be scapegoated. Examples abound, from the Turks in Germany, the Algerians in France, Catholics in Northern Ireland, to the Basques in Spain. The power of national and cultural affiliations is strong. And while the march toward a federalized Europe seems inexorable, popular support, even when it is present, is not overwhelming. What this means for the future is that social cohesion across Europe is threatened, the risk of disintegrating infectious disease control rises, and "blame" will be placed on the shoulders of those already most vulnerable and ostracized.

How Europe distributes its wealth and provides welfare support to the needy and vulnerable will help to define public opinion. Certain tensions will be difficult to surmount. Europe's core of 11 countries that have joined the "euro" (Sweden, Denmark, Greece, and Britain remain outside), with a combined population of 290 million, and accounting for one fifth of the world's gross domestic product, are becoming a single large economy. "Big business" is driving European integration, and business wants cheap labor, lower taxes, smaller welfare states, and freedom of movement of capital. And it is likely those remaining outside the euro will soon be clamoring to join. (For example, Blair is publicly becoming increasingly committed to Europe.) The economic and business disadvantages are just too great to stay outside.

What will happen when some countries grow economically more slowly than others, when unemployment rises more rapidly in one country than another? Will affluent countries support poorer ones, or will they close their borders and insulate themselves from their neighbors' hardships? Social cohesion is threatened by these possibilities. With economic uncertainty rising as workers move across borders with impunity and as the changes in the global market impact, particularly in manufacturing, fascism has started to raise its ugly head again. Nationalism is rising, and in certain pockets the hard right is gaining popularity. This has been seen at both local regional levels and national levels. In recent parliamentary elections, five countries (Austria, Italy, France, Belgium, and Denmark) had hard-right parties that each gained more than 5 percent of the popular vote.[10] In Russia extreme nationalists are gaining support; if they are successful in gaining power, they may threaten the region as a whole.[11] As in the United States, immigrants are being scapegoated for many of society's perceived ills. A forewarning of this has been seen in Germany following reunification, where one consequence was the somewhat unexpected economic hardships felt by many. Many immigrants, particularly Turks, have been vilified, a response in large part sanctioned by Germany's draconian immigration laws (amended only in 1998), where only those with "German blood" had a right to citizenship. It did not matter if you were born in Germany, "if you are born to immigrants, you will die an immigrant. It doesn't matter if you've read Goethe, wear lederhosen and do a Bavarian dance, they'll still treat you like an immigrant."[12] In Britain in late 1998, in a similar vein, a series of articles in national and regional newspapers headlined the threat posed by recent immigrants. The *Daily Mail* headline, "Brutal Crimes of the Asylum Seekers" and an accompanying editorial ("Wolves posing as sacrificial lambs") followed a recent series in the London *Evening Standard* on the same theme. A typical headline was "When 'asylum' means a free pass to paradise."[13] The media can foment nationalist outrage and focus ire on the most vulnerable.

As inequality, uncertainty, and anxiety rise across Europe, as nationalist sentiments and moralizing are given greater voice, and as the tendency to individualize health policy continues, I believe Europeans will all face the questions the United States faced regarding tuberculosis control. How they respond will reflect how far down that road they have gone. If the regions of Europe are no longer the more cohesive units they once were, they shall, I think, respond with a narrowly focused gaze on those at risk of developing tuberculosis, and those infected who threaten the public health.

Although the "deferential nation," England, that economist and essayist Walter Bagehot described no longer exists, the deference to authority, the trust in the benevolence of government and the wisdom of "the Great and the Good" still run through English politics.[14] How Europe will impact on these national characteristics over time is unclear, but many European countries, particularly those in the south and the east, hold those in authority less in awe. As Europe shrinks, as its borders become less defined, skepticism and recalcitrance may replace deference. Europe must learn from the United States. Political transparency must replace paternalistic opacity. And European federalism must devolve authority downward to regions *and* upward to the Union. "European" must have several meanings, not just one. Only if this occurs will any sense of popular "control," of involvement, of influence, of unity, be maintained.

There are, it seems, two choices. Europeans would do well to recall the intention declared at Messina in June 1955, at the inception of the European project. The aim included "the development of common institutions and the progressive fusion of national economies and the progressive harmonisation of their social policies." The political and social institutions of Europe must, therefore, be strengthened, such that social policy (including health and public health policy) and economic policy are strategically directed and coordinated. Cultural antagonisms must be overcome or the consequences of powerful exclusionary forces within protectionist regions must be faced with potentially disastrous consequences for the most vulnerable. We can look to the United States and adopt similar approaches to societies' most vulnerable individuals, or we can consider new approaches that reflect past European successes.

As the economies of the West contract, as the global tuberculosis epidemic continues largely unabated and the threat of drug resistance looms ever larger, will Europeans blame the sick and poor for their dependency and illness? Will coercive measures assume greater prominence as attempts are made to ensure disease control? Or will we move purposefully to redistribute wealth more equitably, advance beyond the rhetoric of equality of opportunity, and integrate and support each other across national and regional boundaries? As borders are more easily transgressed by resistant microorganisms, and as public health programs struggle to maintain control of infectious disease, public health officials may lose public and political credibility through forces beyond their control. They may then, I believe, resort to coercion in an attempt to both maintain control and shore up their credibility. The first flickers of this approach can already be seen.[15] European public health officials have, in 1999, been calling for greater authority to detain non-compliant patients.

Because tuberculosis frequently affects those living on the margins of society, responses to those on the margins may highlight social tensions. Policy responses illuminate social and political mores. In Britain detention of individuals with tuberculosis for prolonged periods is being countenanced, and at a time when there are insufficient community-based programs offering compliance incentives and alternative methods to enhance treatment compliance are inadequately resourced.[16] In 1998 three individuals with tuberculosis in London were issued long detention orders. How legally sound these orders were is open to question; the process of detention certainly offers fewer civil protections than in the United States. There have been suggestions that, as in New York in 1992, the public health legislation should be made clearer.[17] Whether this means that detention becomes dependent on an assessment of compliance, or risk, (and "due process" safeguards introduced) is so far unclear. If the frustration of about 200 physicians and public health doctors at a series of meetings in London in early 1999 is anything to go by, a substantial number of doctors feel greater coercive measures are a necessary part of an effective tuberculosis control program. Ultimately the approach taken with individuals with communicable diseases who are noninfectious but pose a potential public health threat reflects on society itself, the burden citizens are prepared to bear in support of patient autonomy, perceptions of those living on the margins, and commitment to supporting a network of community care for the most vulnerable citizens.

Conclusion

[Selman] Waksman [the discoverer of streptomycin, one of the first effective anti-tuberculosis drugs] and his successors have supplied the world with the weapons with which the eradication of tuberculosis can be accomplished. It would be but a poor return for their brilliance and their dedication if the world, through default, inertia or political maneuvering, were to prove itself incapable of using these weapons to the full.

—Robert Y. Keers,
Pulmonary Tuberculosis: A Journey Down the Centuries, 1978

This book has described the contemporary response of America's greatest city to an epidemic of an ancient, treatable disease, and thereby has described the American social and cultural response to a public health threat that is surrounded by uncertainty. In describing the epidemic and suggesting that recalcitrant, irresponsible behavior can be influenced by society, I have attempted to highlight both the strengths and weaknesses of the U.S. approach to public health. Unless the social forces that encourage recalcitrant behavior are remedied, compliance with treatment, and therefore control of tuberculosis, may remain impossible or at best, very costly. Many of the factors that encourage such antisocial behavior are, perhaps coincidentally, important influences in the causation of disease, and tuberculosis in particular: overcrowding, poverty, inequality, homelessness, a harsh criminal justice system, an inadequate public healthcare system, and policies that produce social isolation and exclusion. This will remain the case, I believe, as long as tuberculosis treatment must be spread over months. Obviously, if a therapeutic vaccine, or "magic bullet," is developed *and* access and provision of this "weapon" is global, then the methods by which control can be achieved may change. But this goal is a long way off and is, quite possibly, not achievable.

I have suggested that the use of coercion should be assessed from a cultural perspective. Obviously, the assessment of, and the lessons learned from, the New York City epidemic are more applicable to Western nations than to less affluent, developing nations, for a number of reasons. The first reason is that the incidence of tuberculosis varies considerably between different countries and in the United States rates are similar to those seen elsewhere in the West. For example, in 1990 the estimated incidence rate of tuberculosis in Western Europe was 23 per 100,000; in Africa it was 191 per 100,000, and in Southeast Asia it was 237 per 100,000.[1] Whereas low tuberculosis rates are prevalent in much of the West, the potential for an epidemic increase that incurs political, public, and public health officials' anxiety is greater than in many developing nations, where high prevalence rates exist and increases fail to generate similar concerns. Differences in baseline prevalence rates help to define the response. Furthermore, the impact of restraining a few potentially dangerous "transmitters" in a high-prevalence region, where most of the populace have already been exposed to *M. tuberculosis,* is less. Moreover, and of great importance, the cost of lengthy patient detention is not negligible and is beyond the health budget of most developing countries. This does not mean that cheaper coercive measures will not be considered, such as isolation in the home, or economic constraints, such as employment restrictions, if anxiety rises, but because of the differences in setting and background prevalence, much of this book is less relevant to developing nations. Yet the moral arguments should still be pertinent.

Second, although "recalcitrance" and noncompliance are not unique to the United States or to Western Europe, cultural and institutional similarities, such as they are, mean that responses to social problems frequently are transposed from one country to another. In the area of crime, for example, "boot camps," the "Three Strikes and You're Out" law, and "teen curfews" for young offenders, and "zero-tolerance" for petty crime, were advocated in Europe after similar approaches had been used in the United States. Likewise "welfare-to-work" for the jobless moved across the Atlantic. This does not mean that willful poor compliance with anti-tuberculosis treatment does not occur in developing countries (despite the assertions of some experts who work for international health organizations) and that approaches used in the West will not work elsewhere. It means that where cultures are similar responses to similar problems may be adopted.

In the case of tuberculosis control in New York City and elsewhere in the United States, we need to ask whether coercion was necessary and if so what it achieved? This chapter explores the use of detention of noninfectious patients as a tool to reduce transmission and as a measure to increase public health officials' credibility.

As was noted in chapter 6, some patients are more likely than others to relapse if they are poorly compliant. Does this mean that, if detention is based on an individualized assessment of the threat posed to public health, some individuals who fail to comply with treatment should be detained while others, in whom the risk of relapse is less despite a similar history of poor compliance, should not? And if so, are such determinations amenable to regulation? It has been suggested that "an externality whose probable impact is restricted to one or a small group does not warrant public action."[2] Adopting this approach suggests that detention should not have been used to control the behavior of a small number of noninfectious patients because the societal costs they posed were so small. Yet as has been pointed out by others, what if the harm that results affects only a few but the consequences are serious?[3] That is, the probability of the event occurring is small, but the magnitude of the impact on any individual or individuals is sizable. This could be the consequence of failing to isolate a homeless tuberculous individual who resided in a shelter with hundreds of others, many of whom are also coinfected with HIV. Although not many would be affected, the consequences to any one individual, particularly if the strain was multidrug resistant, might be catastrophic. Both the burden and the probability should be weighed. A noncompliant individual who is not coinfected with HIV and who has completed, say, three months of treatment poses little threat. Furthermore, if any individual with tuberculosis rarely comes into contact with those most vulnerable to the disease (e.g., children, HIV-infected persons, etc.) and he or she does not complete treatment, then the burden of threat posed to society is probably small.

This issue of public health threat raises a dilemma noted earlier: As the threat to the public declines, should public health police powers wane? How can a scale of legal action be put into practice that responds appropriately to the same behavioral delinquency but has potentially different consequences in different individuals? The answer, surely, is that each case should be assessed anew, with an individualized assessment of risk of relapse (rather than noncompliance); the threat posed to the public should be estimated afresh with each case and in an ongoing manner. Class-based detention is unconstitutional, and detention based on parameters other than public health threat are surely unjust. When the threat to the public is so small that society is prepared to bear that risk, then recourse to detention is not ethically sound. In the case of a noncompliant patient who has completed all but two weeks of treatment, detention is surely unjust if the threat he or she poses is insignificant. How society determines the level of risk it is prepared to bear is another question, but this notion needs to be explicitly recognized. Detention of patients with tuberculosis should be dependent on the threat they pose to the public health and on this concept alone. The use of coercive measures to ensure compliance should not enable the continuation of political inaction on the social causes of recalcitrance. This is not to suggest that those who pose a threat to public health should not be isolated but that isolation of those who do not pose a threat should not provide a smoke screen for political inactivity. From a utilitarian perspective, the trade-off is between the rights of the individual against the benefits that accrue to the population at large. The utility gain across society should be greater than the utility loss to the detainee. What these utilities are and how they are measured is a separate issue, but attempts to define what they are, and determine their magnitude, should be made so that undue burden does not unnecessarily fall on politically expedient individuals.

The English politician Thomas Macaulay recognized more than 100 years ago the dilemma of intrusive government and laissez-faire government.[4] Nowadays neither intrusive paternalistic government nor neglectful impotent government are acceptable in the West (or elsewhere, for that matter). The state is obliged to control certain personal choices in the public interest, but how it does so depends on cultural norms, values, political ideology, pragmatic government, and history. The recent history of tuberculosis control in New York City can be viewed as a reaffirmation of traditional public health methods, and from this perspective public health reasserted its authority. A paternalistic tone, which had declined in force in the 1980s from public health with the advent of HIV, can be felt again, but it lacks concern for the most vulnerable.

It is worth reflecting for a moment on the calls for quarantine regarding HIV, where science and objectivity lent weight to assertions that quarantine was an inappropriate response to curtail transmission. Yale historian David Musto noted some of the complex influences early in the epidemic when he wrote: "The fear of disease . . . arises not just from a reflection on the physiological affects of a pathogen, but from a consideration of the kind of person and habits which are thought to predispose one to the disease. Likewise, quarantine is a response not only to the actual mode of transmission but also to a popular demand to establish a boundary between the kind of persons so diseased and the respectable people who hope to remain healthy."[5] A few years later Columbia-based ethicist Ronald Bayer remarked, again regarding quarantine and HIV: "It was . . . unthinkable that the courts, which had developed such exacting standards for the protection of criminal defendants and which had rejected the unfettered discretion of the state in cases involving the control of juvenile offenders and the commitment of mental patients, would do less in the case of those who might become targets of efforts at isolation and quarantine."[6] Yet, four years later, by 1993, those "exacting standards" have been rejected for tuberculosis, and in the cases of the most vulnerable and alienated in society as Musto might have prophesied

The burden of proof in the civil cases of noninfectious tuberculosis is less exacting than that demanded in criminal cases, and unlike detained mentally ill patients, those with noninfectious tuberculosis are not an immediate danger to others, and the future threat they pose is uncertain. As Tom Frieden, formerly director of the New York Bureau of Tuberculosis Control, commented when referring to the need for greater authority: "We got into a dicey situation where people with just two weeks left to go in their treatment would refuse to take more treatment. We couldn't detain them. I mean, they were smear negative, culture negative and judges would ask us under oath, 'What's the risk of them becoming smear-positive again?'"[7] The answer, of course, would be close to nil. Furthermore, unlike the mentally ill, who could often be accused of "lack[ing] sufficient insight to make a responsible decision,"[8] detention of an individual with tuberculosis outside a mental institution, that is, at the tuberculosis detention unit on Roosevelt Island, implied that the detainee was in a rational state of mind. But a paternalistic approach is less justifiable regarding tuberculosis. Many patients detained have made, it might be argued given their personal circumstances, a "rational" decision. With regard to the frequently used sanction on the mentally ill, that they pose a threat to themselves, the commissioner of health is not authorized to force treatment on a patient who declines to be treated (unless, under mental health provisions the patient is found to be a danger to self *and* lacks insight into his or her condition). Patients with noninfectious tuberculosis threatened with detention lack the rigorous protection through due process afforded those criminally charged and also lack the protection afforded the insane, that of being shown to be a threat to the public. The notion that individuals with tuberculosis identified as specifically dangerous should be detained to a special form of preventive detention whose length is determined by the health commissioner's prediction (and supported by a judge) of what they will do in the future is open to fundamental objection. Where the fallible prediction of future behavior is the determining factor, errors are inevitable and the length of detainees' loss of liberty becomes dependent on mere speculation and conjecture or, more frequently, simply the duration of treatment envisaged. There is the obvious danger that they will be detained unnecessarily when they have ceased to be a threat. This danger is increased if the review process is inadequate, either because it is entrusted to city authorities and/or because representation is poor and no clear guidelines are laid down as to the criteria to be applied.

It has been suggested that with the recognition of AIDS and HIV in the early 1980s, a change occurred in the conceptions of individual and public well-being, a change that contributed to a review of the ethical foundations of healthcare practice. Commentators have implied that as healthcare and public policy responses to HIV and AIDS were formulated, a general consensus emerged against the use of coercive state interventions.[9] But early responses to AIDS and HIV may have been an aberration, a departure from the traditional model of public health practice in which coercion is perceived as a necessary part of the state's public health armamentarium. This was described briefly earlier in relation to the mentally ill and vaccination practices and can be seen now as HIV spreads into different populations, principally poor minorities. Early in the epidemic advocates resisted named-patient (rather than anonymized or coded) reporting and mandatory naming of contacts, unlike what occurs in traditional disease surveillance and notification programs. They argued that confidentiality could not be guaranteed, privacy could not be protected, and coercion would cause people to delay seeking care and thereby transmission might be exacerbated. With health benefits resulting from combination antiretroviral treatment now obvious, and as HIV spreads into poorer, particularly black, populations, calls for named-patient reporting of individuals are again being heard and this time responded to.[10] At the time of this writing 30 states in the United States, most with low or moderate rates of HIV infection, have adopted name reporting. New York, with its high prevalence rate, has recently joined that club. But there is little evidence that named-patient reporting is any more useful than coded anonymized reporting.[11] As long as HIV testing is voluntary, named-patient reporting will remain a poor surveillance tool; its other arguable benefit, of improving access to care, is unproven. Moreover, fears that individuals should be concerned about breeches in confidentiality and may delay being tested when named-patient reporting is used are well founded, so prevention efforts may be harmed.[12] Partner notification, the benefits of which are likewise unclear, is also likely to deter people from seeking to be tested. Although traditional approaches are again being advanced in the area of HIV, evidence of benefit regarding some of these approaches is somewhat lacking, and ideological and political forces, rather than practical public health forces, are weighing heavily in policy determination—public health officials, it could be argued, are regaining lost ground, reasserting their authority. The contemporary response to tuberculosis is part of that movement.

In the arena of HIV, before coercion is used to identify partners exposed to the virus, either sexually or through drug use, it should be clear what the advantages are and how the additional information gained can be used to combat the spread of the virus. Without the provision of care to those found seropositive, and without responding to knowledge we already have about transmission, it may be difficult to persuade persons who resist identifying partners to do so. After all, further surveillance does not tell public health officials how to prevent further spread; that is known already. Surveillance is required to monitor the spread and enable public health efforts to be focused in their responses. Yet without the political will to act on their knowledge, public health officials' enthusiasm for mandatory named-patient reporting and partner notification seems merely to be officialdom getting in the way of action. HIV has not spread in the States because of lack of knowledge regarding modes of transmission, nor through a lack of detailed demographic knowledge of spread (gay men, hemophiliacs, intravenous drug users, and through heterosexual sex). People have known for years how HIV is spread and (especially through *anonymous* seroprevalence surveillance) in which populations it is spreading fastest. Yet despite this knowledge, spread continues faster in the United States than most Western nations, particularly among poor minority populations. Why? Because approaches to curtail disease spread have not been as aggressively pursued as elsewhere. The debates over sex education, condom advertising, and expansion of needle exchanges have largely been settled elsewhere but continue to rage in the United States. The public health benefits of such programs are clear. "Politics" stymies a strategic response and interferes with coordinated action. It is moral delicacy, not lack of epidemiological knowledge, that has failed to halt HIV spread in the United States. Yet now, in seeking to prevent spread to "innocent spouses," law makers in New York and elsewhere are requiring people who seek treatment for HIV to provide the names of sexual and drug-using contacts.

The period when the role of education is stressed relative to regulatory measures may be passing. Health officials' hope to foster personal responsibility through education and social support is fading. Ironically, this has happened in New York despite the concerns about "big government" intervention and while a Republican governor is incumbent in the state house and a Republican mayor sits in city hall. Government interference is not dead, it just, as always, wears a "moral" hat.

Regarding tuberculosis control in New York City, detention played a crucial role, as Frieden and others in the Bureau of Tuberculosis Control acknowledge, in public health officials' attempts to regain credibility among their clinical colleagues. The chaos of the public health service and the urgency of action that the epidemic demanded meant that, for the bureau to respond in anything like a coordinated fashion, physicians needed to believe the city "meant business." In practice, when physicians called the bureau about a patient who would not comply with treatment, the bureau had to respond in a meaningful way that the clinicians could understand. The alternative was that doctors would simply bypass the service and react to problems as they came through the emergency room doors, the "revolving doors" through which patients who had been discharged weeks before returned having relapsed for the fourth or fifth time. The bureau needed to regain credibility, and fast. Detention achieved this aim. It appealed to clinicians because they would no longer have to deal with delinquent patients whose treatment was becoming more and more complex as they developed strains of tuberculosis resistant to ever more drugs; it appealed to healthcare organizations as they could move disruptive, unprofitable patients on to other facilities; and it appealed to the public and politicians because it smacked of a firm response to what was viewed as a frightening threat.

Detention also allowed public health officials to regain credibility with their patients. Certainly patients could no longer thumb their noses at their doctors and refuse to take their medication, or at least not with the same impunity. But, as most in the bureau acknowledge, patients who do so are only a small minority. Most patients simply needed a better organized service that provided care to them and assisted them, that was not a bureaucratic time-wasting minefield where care provision was erratic at best. The bureau gained credibility with these patients by providing an appropriate service. The extent the undercurrent of coercion, the background threat, had on the doctor-patient relationship has not been examined. But the relationship will have been changed as a consequence, with the authority of the doctor enhanced and an element of fear introduced.

From a multicausal and social perspective, tuberculosis is caused by poverty, overcrowding, malnutrition, and social inequity. It is a measure of social justice, hence its fascination. From a "germ theory" perspective, its cause is, obviously, the organism *M. tuberculosis,* and health is influenced by its interaction with other microorganisms, particularly HIV. In extending this biomedical model, genetic influences, where they have been elucidated, also gain increasing authority.[13] But even when this narrow biomedical model is accepted in toto, social forces still can be seen to influence its transmission, the clinical picture, and response to treatment. Drugs must be given to treat patients and transmission must be curtailed; doing this effectively requires effective surveillance, early diagnosis, and effective management of the disease with good access to healthcare. The tangle of biomedical and social influencing factors may be impossible to unravel.

Yet a biomedical individualized approach that pays scant attention to the social causes of tuberculosis is often more acceptable to policy-makers. It appears "tight" and there are no "loose ends." The complex network of influences can be distilled such that a single node in that network is seen as the problem and other nodes can be disregarded. In this regard, the noncompliant individual is seen as the issue that needs redressing rather than the milieu in which those most susceptible to tuberculosis as well as those who were noncompliant flourished. This is an appealing approach. One can focus policy and measure the effects of intervention. This "focused" approach is reflected in medicine's over-whelming emphasis on molecular and pharmacological approaches to disease, the "magic bullet" cures. Despite being clearly documented, the complicated interactions of society on disease are largely ignored. Compared to the West's vast expenditure on medical care and biomedi-cal research, public health spending is tiny, and efforts to remedy societal inequities often are ineffectual or unacceptable. This biomedical approach to the causal chain of disease was described by political scientist Sylvia Tesh in her book *Hidden Arguments*.[14] She suggests that, after microorganisms, personal behavior is recognized as an intermediate cause of disease, environmental pollution is a tertiary cause, and only at the very end of the chain are sociopolitical realities emphasized. The West concentrates its resources on the first cause; only when this is unsuccessful does the second cause receive attention; and so on. In tuberculosis control, this approach can be seen such that, although effective drugs have been available for decades, their promise has not been recognized and now behavioral modification is receiving attention through directly observed therapy programs. The sociopolitical causes have yet to be addressed.

As Tesh notes, such an approach "makes logical the idea that the most efficient method of disease prevention provides the individual human body with a way to fight invasions of microscopic particles, and it expands to advocate behavioral change only when no such particles have been identified. Changing the physical environment is, from this perspective, a third choice, and to attack poverty as a way to reduce disease becomes a last resort." Although, obviously, the microorganism that causes tuberculosis has been identified, her sentiments still hold true because, since the microbiological approach has not lived up to its initial promise, emphasis has shifted to personal behavior. Redressing the social causes of tuberculosis, although often given lipservice, receives little attention. In New York what enthusiasm there was soon waned after tuberculosis returned to its traditional stronghold, immigrants, the homeless, and those infected with HIV, and drug-resistant strains stopped threatening the wider population.

The reason this multicausal approach to disease has not gained policymakers' attention is, in large part, not because of expense (the usual excuse) but because of difficulties in determining the precise cost and effect of interventions. Public health policy, like most social policy, is often invisible, and its successes are not easily quantifiable. Yet, as Margaret Hamburg noted while commissioner of health in New York City: "It is increasingly clear that the burden of illness will not yield to exclusively medical solutions, yet many of the casualties land on the doorstep of the healthcare delivery system."[15] It has been easier politically to concentrate on cure rather than prevention. Another of the drawbacks to this wider societal approach is that there is an implicit belief that policies will, necessarily, be inefficient and too slow. Certainly, in an emergency, such as the New York City epidemic, focused public health initiatives are necessary and probably cost effective. Yet to be truly effective over the long term, tuberculosis control policies must focus on the fundamental social causes that give rise to the disease and aggravate its spread *and* give emphasis to the microorganism.

What determines policy choices is, in many cases, the wrong question. The question that received the most political attention when New York City faced an epidemic of resistant strains of an age-old scourge was: "Who fails to comply with antituberculous treatment and what can be done to ensure they comply?" not "Why do large numbers of individuals with tuberculosis fail to adhere to treatment?" With regard to the concentration of tuberculosis cases in large cities, the question should be not so much "Who gets tuberculosis in the city?" but rather "Why is this disease, a disease of poverty and overcrowding, increasing in incidence in one of the most affluent cities on earth?" With regard to the overall excess mortality in poor inner city areas Colin McCord and Harold Freeman, whose paper appeared in the *New England Journal of Medicine,* suggested that "special consideration analogous to that given to natural-disaster areas" is justified.[16] Yet the documented increases in mortality rates in Harlem have not resulted from of a freak of nature; the relationship between early death and the environment was not merely stochastic. But the response suggests it was.

Structural and political interventions are rarely considered and, when they are, receive less attention. Better healthcare provision and behavioral change are the answers emphasized. As ethicist Alan Garfinkel noted, the difference is between asking an individualistic question and a structural question.[17] The individualistic question demands an individualized answer (and policy response), which is simpler than the structural question, which may demand institutional and societal reform. The answer depends on the question. In the United States, and increasingly in Europe, individualistic questions are sometimes the only ones given consideration.

Cultural differences dictate responses to events. Politicians can respond, but they need popular support. The "Tear Drop" campaign that resulted from the shooting of several small school children in Dunblane, Scotland on March 13, 1996, rapidly resulted in political pressure and consequently handguns being banned. The question asked was not so much "Why did *he,* the perpetrator, do this?" or "How can we identify such people in the future?" (both of which are largely unanswerable) but "How can society prevent this from occurring again?" Emphasis on the first question is more representative of an individualized societal response common in the United States where a spate of children with firearms killing other children in schools recently occurred. "Why do *these* children kill?" is the focus. Few have asked the structural question: "How can we stop children who want to kill, those who are all but impossible to identify before the act, from carrying out these awful deeds?"

To be fair, occasionally structural questions are asked, the problem is that an effective political response has not received enough support. Therefore, the problem is not only that the structural questions are not asked but that, when they are, policy responses are insufficiently supported. Politicians are impotent without a mandate. The U.S. response to children carrying guns has concentrated on the motives of the perpetrators and the detection of others predisposed to such deeds—a germ theory/ personal behavior approach rather than a societal approach. How many children need to die at the hands of other children with firearms before the structural question is seriously addressed? How bad does the excess mortality in Harlem need to get before the structural questions are asked? The answers to these questions are obviously more, and worse.

In 1981 social scientists Leon Eisenberg and Arthur Kleinman attempted to define a better relationship between the social sciences and medicine when they suggested: "The key task for medicine is not to diminish the role of the biomedical sciences in the theory and practice of medicine but to supplement them with an equal application of the social sciences in order to provide both a more comprehensive understanding of disease and better care of the patient. The problem is not 'too much science,' but too narrow a view of the sciences relevant to medicine."[18] They were not suggesting that the biomedical model should be rejected, simply that account should be taken of societal influences and that overemphasis on individuality in response to a disease neglects a broader and quite possibly more cost-effective and certainly more just approach. Nearly 20 years later we are farther away than ever from that goal. The fact that a more just approach requires political authority does not negate its appeal or the strength of the argument. Ultimately the burden of responding to the real questions should fall on elected public servants. Because the questions are difficult does not mean they should not be asked. But because they are difficult may mean they will not be acknowledged and probably will not be answered.

What is needed is political will instilled by a populace moved to demand action and a political mandate for government. This depends on articulate debate regarding government's interventionist role, not sloganizing about "Big Government," a national recognition that inequities exist and should be remedied, and leadership and policies to enhance social cohesion rather than divide the deserving from the undeserving. In essence, the right questions need to be asked, answers demanded, and states and substate regions moved to action. It must be recognized that the narrow biomedical approach is politically useful, politically neutral, and encourages the view that society need not be changed, that social intervention is unnecessary. To control tuberculosis we must fashion policies that are just, care indiscriminately for those who fall ill, are cognizant of cultural context, are responsive to societal needs, and are not simply a means to reassert credibility. Policy must be subverted neither by those who, through fear and anxiety, demand overly coercive measures, nor by those who fail to recognize any personal accountability and see nothing wrong in posing a threat to others. The history of earlier responses to infectious diseases serves as a warning to the folly of unnecessarily draconian measures, but likewise, a laissez-faire attitude may also reap appalling rewards. The United States and, in the future, Europe, should be candid about the policies being adopted. A society that cares for, helps, and treats the vulnerable, rather than punishes, confines, and controls them needs to be established. Just as the benefits individuals with tuberculosis accrue through measures to enhance treatment compliance should be explicit, so too should self-interested paternalism be recognized for what it is. Coercion, as a tool in the public health armamentarium, is here to stay, but it should be used sparingly, with appropriate attention to due process legal doctrines, and only where a significant threat to the public health is posed.

APPENDIX

NEW YORK CITY HEALTH CODE:
AMENDMENTS TO 11.47, SUBSECTION (E) TO (J)

Subsection (e) set out the procedural framework relating to (d), whereby authority is exercised and, in addition, established that the burden of proof is on the commissioner and requires the commissioner to "prove the particularized circumstances constituting the necessity for such detention by clear convincing evidence."

Subsection (f), again pursuant to (d), set out what facts and notice must be given to the person being detained. It set forth that "an individualized assessment of the person's circumstances and/or behavior constituting the basis for the issuance of such order" is given and that "the less restrictive alternatives that were attempted and were unsuccessful and/or the less restrictive treatment alternatives that were considered and rejected, and the reasons such alternatives were rejected are given."

Subsection (g) set out the events whereby detention would be terminated automatically; for example, a person who is detained solely because he or she is infectious and cannot be properly isolated so as to prevent others becoming infected must be released when no longer infectious, or "after the Department ascertains that changed circumstances exist that permit him or her to be adequately separated from others" so that the person, although infectious, will be adequately separated from others while infectious.

Subsections (h) and (i) require the provision of interpreters and make it clear that forcible administration of medication is not authorized, respectively.

Subsection (j) defines the term "active tuberculosis." It exists where there has been (a) a positive smear or culture taken from a pulmonary or laryngeal source and the patient has not completed a course of treatment for tuberculosis, or (b) where "a positive smear or culture from an extra-pulmonary source has tested positive for tuberculosis and there is clinical evidence or clinical suspicion of pulmonary tuberculosis disease and the person has not completed an appropriate prescribed course of medication for tuberculosis." Or (c) "in those cases where sputum smears or cultures are unobtainable, the radiographic evidence, in addition to current clinical evidence and/or laboratory tests, is sufficient to establish a medical diagnosis of pulmonary tuberculosis." Patients with active tuberculosis are considered infectious until three consecutive sputum smears collected on separate days are negative "and the clinical symptoms of tuberculosis have resolved or significantly improved."

NOTES

CHAPTER 1

1. K. A. Sepkowitz, E. E. Telzak, S. Recalde, and D. Armstrong. "Trends in Susceptibility of Tuberculosis in New York City, 1987-1991." *Clinical Infectious Disease* 18, no. 75 (1994): 5-9; T. R. Frieden, T. Sterling, A. Pablos-Mendez, J. O. Kilbum, G. M. Cauthen, and S. W. Dooley. "The Emergence of Drug-Resistant Tuberculosis in New York City." *New England Journal of Medicine* 3, no. 328 (1993): 521-26.

2. S. E. Valway, R. B. Grelfinger, M. Papania, et al. "Multidrug-Resistant Tuberculosis in the New York State Prison System, 1990-1991." *Journal of Infectious Disease,* no. 170 (1994): 151-56; T. R. Frieden, L. F. Sherman, K. L. Maw, et al. "A Multi-Institutional Outbreak of Highly Drug-Resistant Tuberculosis." *Journal of the American Medical Association* 276 (1996): 1229-35; T. R. Frieden, C. L. Woodley, J. T. Crawford, D. Lew, and S. M. Dooley. "The Molecular Epidemiology of Tuberculosis in New York City: The Importance of Nosocomial Transmission and Laboratory Error." *Tubercle and Lung Disease* 77 (1996): 407-13.

3. New York City, NY, Health Code 11.55 (1993).

4. "Outbreak of Hospital Acquired Multidrug Resistant Tuberculosis." *Communicable Disease Report* 5, no. 34 (1995): 161.

5. P. Mayho. *The Tuberculosis Survival Handbook.* London: XLR8, 1999.

6. Ibid.

7. R. J. Coker. "Uncertainty, Civil Liberties, Coercion, and Public Health." *British Medical Journal* 318 (1999): 1434-35.

8. S. Sontag. Illness as Metaphor; and, AIDS and Its Metaphors. New York: Anchor Books, Doubleday, 1990.

9. T. Dormandy. The White Death: A History of Tuberculosis. London: The Hambledon Press, 1999.

10. E. Sumartojo. "When Tuberculosis Treatment Fails: A Social Behavioural Account of Patient Adherence." *American Review of Respiratory Disease* 147 (1993): 1311-20; *From Compliance to Concordance: Achieving Shared Goals in Medicine Taking.* London: Royal Pharmaceutical Society of Great Britain, 1997.

11. C. H. Foreman Jr. *Plagues, Products & Politics: Emergent Public Health Hazards and National Policymaking.* Washington, DC: The Brookings Institution, 1994.

12. S. E. Weis, P. C. Slocum, F. X. Blais, et al. "The Effect of Directly Observed Therapy on the Rates of Drug Resistance and Relapse in Tuberculosis. *New*

England Journal of Medicine 330 (1994): 1179-84; C. P. Chaulk, K. Moore-Rice, R. T. Rizzo, R. E. Chaisson. "Eleven Years of Community-based Directly Observed Therapy for Tuberculosis." *Journal of the American Medical Association* 274 (1995): 945-51.

13. Advisory Council for the Elimination of Tuberculosis. "Initial Therapy for Tuberculosis in the Era of Multidrug Resistance: Recommendations of the Advisory Council for the Elimination of Tuberculosis." *Morbidity and Mortality Weekly Report* 42, no. RR/7 (1993); American Thoracic Society, Centers for Disease Control and Prevention, American Academy of Pediatrics, Infectious Disease Society of America. "Control of Tuberculosis in the United States." *American Review of Respiratory Disease* 146 (1992): 1623-33.

14. R. Bayer and D. Wilkinson. "Directly Observed Therapy for Tuberculosis: History of an Idea." *Lancet* 345 (1995): 1545; C. P. Chaulk and D. S. Pope. "The Baltimore City Health Department Program of Directly Observed Therapy for Tuberculosis." *Clinics in Chest Medicine* 18 (1997): 149-54.

15. M. D. Iseman, D. L. Cohn, and J. A. Sbarbaro. "Directly Observed Treatment of Tuberculosis: We Can't Afford Not to Try It." *New England Journal of Medicine* 328 (1993): 576-78.

16. Weis et al., "Effect of Directly Observed Therapy on the Rates of Drug Resistance and Relapse in Tuberculosis"; W. J. Burman, C. B. Dalton, D. L. Cohn, J. R. G. Butler, and R. R. Reves. "A Cost-Effectiveness Analysis of Directly Observed Therapy vs. Self-Administered Therapy for Treatment of Tuberculosis." *Chest* 112 (1997): 63-70.

17. A. Pablos-Mendez, M. C. Raviglione, A. Laszlo, et al. "Global Surveillance for Antituberculosis-Drug Resistance, 1994-1997." *New England Journal of Medicine* 338 (1998): 1641-49.

18. Ibid.; J. M. Watson. "Results of a National Survey of Tuberculosis Notifications in England and Wales in 1993." *Thorax* 50 (1995): 442P.

19. T. Moulding, A. K. Dutt, and L. B. Reichman. "Fixed Combinations of Antituberculous Medications to Prevent Drug Resistance. *Annals of Internal Medicine* 122 (1995): 951-54.

20. Bayer and Wilkinson, "Directly Observed Therapy for Tuberculosis."

21. R. Bayer, C. Stayton, M. Desvarieux, C. Healton, S. Landesman, and W. Tsai. "Directly Observed Therapy and Treatment Completion for Tuberculosis in the United States: Is Universal Supervised Therapy Necessary?" *American Journal of Public Health* 88, no. 7 (1998): 1052-58.

22. M. Zwarenstein, J. H. Schoeman, C. Vundule, C. J. Lombard, and M. Tatley. "Randomised Controlled Trial of Self-Supervised and Directly Observed Treatment of Tuberculosis." *Lancet* 352 (1998): 1340-43.

23. T. A. Kenyon, M. J. Mwasekaga, R. Huebner, D. Rumisha, N. Binkin, and E. Maganu. "Low Levels of Drug Resistance Amidst Rapidly Increasing Tuberculosis and Human Immunodeficiency Virus Co-epidemics in Botswana." *International Journal of Tuberculosis and Lung Disease* 3 (1999): 4-11.

24. Bayer et al., "Directly Observed Therapy and Treatment Completion for Tuberculosis in the United States."

25. Singapore Tuberculosis Service/British Medical Research Council. "Assessment of a Daily Combined Preparation of Isoniazid, Rifampin and Pyrazinamide in a Controlled Trial of Three 6-month Regimens for Smear-Positive

Pulmonary Tuberculosis." *American Review of Respiratory Disease* 143 (1991): 707-12; Hong Kong Chest Service/British Medical Research Council. "Controlled Trial of 2, 4 and 6 Months Pyrazinamide in 6-month, Three-Times-Weekly Regimens for Smear-Positive Pulmonary Tuberculosis, Including an Assessment of a Combined Preparation of Isoniazid, Rifampicin, and Pyrazinamide. Results at 30 Months." *American Review of Respiratory Disease* 143 (1991): 700-6; L. J. Geiter, R. J. O'Brien, D. L. Combs, and D. E. Snider Jr. "United States Public Health Service Tuberculosis Therapy Trial 21: Preliminary Results of an Evaluation of a Combination Tablet of Isoniazid, Rifampicin and Pyrazinamide." *Tubercle* 68 (1987): 41-46; D. L. Combs, R. J. O'Brien, and L. J. Geiter. "USPHS Tuberculosis Short-Course Chemotherapy Study Trial 21: Effectiveness, Toxicity, and Acceptability. The Report of Final Results." *Annals of Internal Medicine* 112, no. 3 (1990): 97-406.

26. Ibid.

27. Ibid.

28. Hong Kong Chest Service/British Medical Research Council. "Controlled Trial of 2, 4 and 6 Months Pyrazinamide"; Geiter et al., "United States Public Health Service Tuberculosis Therapy Trial 21"; and Combs, O'Brien, and Geiter. "USPHS Tuberculosis Short-Course Chemotherapy Study Trial 21."

29. Hong Kong Chest Service/British Medical Research Council. "Controlled Trial of 2, 4 and 6 Months Pyrazinamide."

30. Zwarenstein et al., "Randomised Controlled Trial of Self-Supervised and Directly Observed Treatment of Tuberculosis."

31. R. D. Moore, C. P. Chaulk, R. Griffiths, S. Cavalcante, and R. Chaisson. "Cost- Effectiveness of Directly Observed versus Self-Administered Therapy for Tuberculosis." *American Journal of Respiratory and Critical Care Medicine* 154 (1996): 1013-19.

32. "Tuberculosis." City Health Information (New York) 15, no. 4 (1996): 12-13; K. Brudney and J. Dobkin. "Resurgent Tuberculosis in New York City: Human Immunodeficiency Virus, Homelessness and the Decline of Tuberculosis Control Programmes." *American Review of Respiratory Disease* 144 (1991): 745-49.

CHAPTER 2

1. R. J. Coker. "Lessons from New York's Tuberculosis Epidemic: Tuberculosis Is a Political as Much as a Medical Problem and So Are the Solutions." *British Medical Journal* 317 (1998): 616.

2. G. Rosen. "The Bacteriologic, Immunologic and Chemotherapeutic Period, 1875-1950." *Bulletin of the New York Academy of Medicine* 40 (1964): 483-94.

3. A. Lucksted and R. D. Coursey. "Consumer Perceptions of Pressure and Force in Psychiatric Treatments." *Psychiatric Services* 46 (1995): 146-52.

4. G. Feldman, personal communication, 1997.

5. F. Allport. "The J-Curve Hypothesis of Conforming Behaviour." *Journal of Social Psychology* 5 (1934): 141-83.

6. W. L. Atkinson, S. C. Hadler, S. B. Redd, and W. A. Orenstein. "Measles Surveillance—United States, 1991." *Morbidity and Mortality Weekly Report* 41 (SS-6) (1992): 1-12.

7. R. H. Bernier "Assessment of Immunization Coverage: A Critical Element in The Strategy to Reach 90 Percent Levels." In: *25th National Immunization Conference Proceedings,* June 10-13, 1991, Washington, DC. Atlanta

8. Centers for Disease Control. "Retrospective Assessment of Vaccination Coverage among School-aged Children—Selected U.S. Cities." *Morbidity and Mortality Weekly Report* 41 (1992): 103-7.

9. COVER/Korner: July to September 1998. "Vaccination Coverage Statistics for Children Up to 5 Years of Age in the United Kingdom." *Communicable Disease Report* 9, no. 5 (1999): 39-40.

10. H. M. Leichter. *Free To Be Foolish: Politics and Health Promotion in the United States and Great Britain.* Princeton, NJ: Princeton University Press, 1991.

11. F. P. Grad. *The Public Health Law Manual* (2nd ed.). Washington, DC: American Public Health Association, 1990.

12. D. Porter and R. Porter. "The Enforcement of Health: The British Debate." In: E. Fee and D. M. Fox, eds., *AIDS: The Burdens of History.* Berkeley: University of California Press, 1988: 97-120.

13. B. J. Stern, ed. *Should We Be Vaccinated?* New York: Harper & Brothers, 1927.

14. "Vaccination, the Largest Question of the Day." *Vaccination Tracts,* no. 14 (1879).

15. G. Gibbs. "Evils of Vaccination." In: B. J. Stern, ed. *Should We Be Vaccinated?* New York: Harper & Brothers. 1927.

16. D. Roberts. *Paternalism in Early Victorian England.* London: Croom Helm, 1979.

17. R. M. Macleod. "Law, Medicine and Public Opinion: The Resistance to Compulsory Health Legislation, 1870-1907." *Public Law* 107 (1967): 189-211.

18. Public Health (Infectious Diseases) Regulations. 1988.

19. COVER/Korner, "Vaccination Coverage Statistics for Children Up to 5 Years of Age in the United Kingdom."

20. Stern, ed., *Should We Be Vaccinated?*

21. *Jacobson v. Massachusetts,* 197 U.S. 11 (1905).

22. Ibid.

23. Stern, ed., *Should We Be Vaccinated?*

24. Grad, *Public Health Law Manual.*

25. W. Schumacher. "Legal/Ethical Aspects of Vaccinations." *Developments in Biological Standardization* 43 (1979): 435-38.

26. W. Gaylin and B. Jenings. *The Perversion of Autonomy: The Proper Uses of Coercion and Constraints in a Liberal Society.* New York: The Free Press, 1996.

27. J. Q. La Fond and M. L. Durham. *Back to the Asylum: The Future of Mental Health Law and Policy in the United States.* New York: Oxford University Press, 1992.

28. Ibid.

29. G. Grob. *Mental Illness and American Society.* Princeton, NJ: Princeton University Press, 1983.

30. C. A. Kiesler and A. E. Sibulkin. *Mental Hospitalization: Myths and Facts about a National Crisis.* Beverly Hills, CA: Sage Publications, 1987.

31. E. Goffman. *Asylums.* New York: Doubleday, 1961; Joint Commission on Mental Illness and Health. *Action for Mental Health.* New York: Basic Books, 1961.

32. La Fond and Durham. *Back to the Asylum.*
33. *Lessard v. Schmidt,* 349 F. Supp. 1078 (E. D. Wis. 1972).
34. *Addington v. Texas,* 441 U.S. 418, 427 (1979); *Suzuki v. Yuen,* 438 F. Supp. 1106 (D. Haw. 1977); In re Powell, 85 111. App. 3d 877, 879-80, 407 N. E.2d 658, 660 (1980).
35. *O'Connor v. Donaldson,* 422 U.S. 563, 575 (1975).
36. *Colyar v. Third Judicial District Court,* 469 F. Supp. 424 (D. Utah 1979).
37. La Fond and Durham. *Back to the Asylum.*
38. N. Rhoden. "The Limits of Liberty: Deinstitutionalization, Homelessness, and Libertarian Theory." *Emory Law Journal* 31, no. 2 (1982): 375-440.
39. La Fond and Durham. *Back to the Asylum.*
40. F. Butterfield. "Treatment Can Be Illusion for Violent Mentally Ill." *New York Times,* July 28, 1998: Al, A12.
41. D. L. Dennis and J. Monahan, eds. *Coercion and Aggressive Community Treatment: A New Frontier in Mental Health Law.* New York: Plenum Press, 1996.
42. *Greene v. Edwards,* 263 S. E. 2d 661, 662 (W. Va 1980).
43. C. E. Rosenberg. *The Cholera Years.* Chicago: University of Chicago Press, 1962.
44. G. Rosen. *A History of Public Health.* New York: MD Publications, 1958.
45. "Second Annual Report of the Metropolitan Board of Health of the State of New York, 1867." New York, 1868.
46. P. Starr. *The Social Transformation of American Medicine.* New York: Basic Books, 1982.
47. H. Biggs. "The Registration of Tuberculosis." *The Philadelphia Medical Journal,* December 1, 1900: 1023-29.
48. Ibid.; C.-E. A. Winslow. *The Life of Hermann Biggs.* Philadelphia: Lea and Febiger, 1929.
49. Winslow. *The Life of Hermann Biggs.*
50. D. M. Fox. "Social Policy and City Politics: Tuberculosis Reporting in New York, 1889-1900. *Bulletin of the History of Medicine* 49 (1975): 169-95.
51. C. A. Wilson. *The Contributions of Hermann Biggs to Public Health.* New York: 1928.
52. S. H. Adams. "Tuberculosis: The Real Race Suicide." *McClure's* 24 (1905): 234-49.
53. "Society Report: Philadelphia County Medical Society." *The Philadelphia Medical Journal,* December 1, 1900: 1010-12.
54. Ibid.
55. Request to Amend Section 11.47 Health Code. From Kenneth Ong, Deputy Commissioner of Disease Intervention to Margaret Hamburg, Commissioner of Health, New York City. October 6, 1992.
56. C. V. Chapin. "History of State and Municipal Control of Disease." In: M. P. Ravenal, ed. *A Half Century of Public Health.* New York: American Public Health Association, 1921:135-37.
57. *Papers of Charles V. Chapin, M.D.* New York: The Commonwealth Fund, 1934.
58. J. H. Cassedy. *Charles V. Chapin and the Public Health Movement.* Cambridge, MA: Harvard University Press, 1962; E. L. Trudeau. "Environment in Its

Relation to the Progress of Bacterial Invasion in Tuberculosis." *Transactions of the American Climatological Association* 4 (1887): 131-36.

59. S. A. Knopf. *Tuberculosis as a Disease of the Masses and How to Combat It* (4th ed.). New York: Fred P. Flori, 1907.

60. Trudeau, "Environment in its Relation to the Progress of Bacterial Invasion in Tuberculosis."

61. "Second Annual Report of the Metropolitan Board of Health."

62. "Annual Report. New York: New York City Department of Health, 1895.

63. H. Biggs. "To Rob Consumption of Its Terrors." *The Forum* 16 (1894): 767.

64. Winslow, *The Life of Hermann Biggs.*

65. Papers of Charles V. Chapin, M.D.

66. G. B. Webb and D. S. Powell. *Henry Sewall, Physiologist and Physician.* Baltimore: Johns Hopkins University Press, 1946.

67. C. W. Ingraham. "Control of Tuberculosis from a Strictly Medico-Legal Standpoint." *Journal of the American Medical Association,* September 28, 1896: 694.

68. W. Welch. Address to the fifth meeting of the National Association for the Study and Prevention of Disease. *Transactions,* 1909: 36.

69. J. A. Tobey. *Public Health Law,* 3rd ed. New York: The Commonwealth Fund, 1947.

70. W. H. Conley. "Detention of Consumptives in a City Hospital." *Journal of the Outdoor Life* 11 (1914): 104.

71. S. M. Rothman. "Seek and Hide: Public Health Departments and Persons with Tuberculosis, 1890-1940." *Journal of Law, Medicine and Ethics* 21, nos. 3-4 (1993): 289-95.

72. Wilson RJ. Difficulties encountered by hospital authorities in detaining homeless consumptives. *Journal of the Outdoor Life* 1914; 11: 102.

73. Committee on Hospitals for Advanced Cases of Tuberculosis. "Report." *Transactions of the Ninth Annual Meeting of the National Association for the Study and Prevention of Tuberculosis* 1913: 54-66.

74. Rothman. "Seek and Hide"; S. M. Rothman. *Living in the Shadow of Death: Tuberculosis and the Social Experience of Illness in American History.* Baltimore: The Johns Hopkins University Press, 1995.

75. M. M. Davis and M. C. Jarrett. *A Health Inventory of New York City.* New York: Welfare Council of New York City, 1929.

76. *New York Times,* March 3, 1937: Quoted in Rosen. *A History of Public Health.*

77. J. H. Emerson. *Collected Works of Haven Emerson.* New York: 1962, vol. 3.

78. *Annual Report.* New York: Board of Health, 1937.

79. R. C. Williams. *The United States Public Health Service.* Washington, DC: Commissioned Officers Association of the United States Public Health Service, 1951.

80. D. Widelock, L. R. Peizer, and S. Klein. "Public Health Significance of *Tubercle* Bacilli Resistant to Isoniazid." *American Journal of Public Health* 45 (1955): 79-83.

81. C. Northrop, J. H. Fountain, and D. W. Zahn. "The Practical Management of the Recalcitrant Tuberculous Patient." *Public Health Reports* 67 (1952): 895-86.

82. B. E. Lerner. "On What Authority Is This Being Done? Tuberculosis

Control, Poverty and Coercion in Seattle, 1909-1973." Ph.D. diss. Seattle: University of Washington, 1996.

83. L. Baumgartner. "Urban Reservoirs of Tuberculosis." *American Review of Tuberculosis* 79 (1959):687-89.

84. *Annual Report.* New York: New York City Department of Health, 1959-60. *Annual Report.* New York: Board of Health, 1961-62.

85. *Annual Report,* 1961-62.

86. G. James. "Fragmentation: Crucial Flaw in the Health Care Complex." *Hospitals* 38 (1964): 28-31.

87. *Annual Report.* New York: Board of Health, 1965-66.

88. P. Aswapokee, N. Aswapokee, C. Ortiz-Neu, P. D. Ellner, and H. C. Neu. "Drug-Resistant Tuberculosis: Serious Problem." *New York State Journal of Medicine* 80 (1980): 1541-45.

89. *Tuberculosis in New York City, 1970: A Report to the Mayor and the Citizens of the City of New York.* New York: Tuberculosis and Respiratory Disease Association of New York, 1971.

CHAPTER 3

1. K. Brudney and J. Dobkin. "A Tale of Two Cities: Tuberculosis Control in Managua and New York City." *Seminars in Respiratory Infections* 6 (1991): 261-72.

2. ATS. "Control of Tuberculosis in the United States." *American Review of Respiratory Disease* 146 (1992): 1623-33.

3. *Tuberculosis in New York City, 1989.* New York: New York City Department of Health, Bureau of Tuberculosis Control, 1989.

4. K. Brudney and J. Dobkin. "Resurgent Tuberculosis in New York City: Human Immunodeficiency Virus, Homelessness and the Decline of Tuberculosis Control Programmes." *American Review of Respiratory Disease* 144 (1991): 745-49.

5. J. W. Pape, B. Liautaud, F. Thomas, et al. "Characteristics of the Acquired Immunodeficiency Syndrome (AIDS) in Haiti." *New England Journal of Medicine* 309 (1983): 945-50; G. Sunderam, R. J. McDonald, T. Maniatis, J. Oleske, R. Kapila, and L. B. Reichnian. "Tuberculosis as a Manifestation of the Acquired Immunodeficiency Syndrome (AIDS)." *Journal of the American Medical Association* 256 (1986): 362-66.

6. P. S. Arno, C. J. L. Murray, K. A. Bonuck, and P. Alcabes. "The Economic Impact of Tuberculosis in Hospitals in New York City: A Preliminary Analysis." *Journal of Law, Medicine, and Ethics* 21, nos. 3-4 (1993): 317-23.

7. D. L. Morse, B. I. Truman, J. P. Hanrahan, et al. "AIDS behind Bars. Epidemiology of New York State Prison Inmate Cases, 1980-1988." *New York State Journal of Medicine* 90 (1990): 133-38.

8. M. M. Braun, B. I. Truman, B. Maguire, et al. "Increasing Incidence of Tuberculosis in a Prison Inmate Population: Association with HIV Infection." *Journal of the American Medical Association* 261, no. 3 (1989): 393-97.

9. P. Alcabes, P. Vossenas, R. Cohen, C. Braslow, D. Michaels, and S. Zoloth. "Compliance with Isoniazid Prophylaxis in Jail." *American Review of Respiratory Disease* 140 (1989): 1194-97.

10. *Tuberculosis in New York City, 1991.* New York City Department of Health, Bureau of Tuberculosis Control, 1991.

11. M. N. Sherman, M. S. Brickner, and M. S. Schwartz. "Tuberculosis in Single-Room Occupancy Hotel Residents: A Persisting Focus of Disease." *New York Medical Journal* 2 (1980): 39-41.

12. P. W. Brickner, L. K. Scharer, B. A. Conanan, M. Savarese, and B. C. Scanlan, eds. *Under the Safety Net: The Health and Social Welfare of the Homeless in the United States.* New York: W. W. Norton & Co., 1992; *Tuberculosis in New York City, 1984-1985.* New York: New York City Department of Health: 1987.

13. *Tuberculosis in New York City, 1992.* New York: New York City Department of Health, 1992.

14. J. M. McAdam, P. W. Brickner, L. L. Scharer, J. A. Crocco, and A. E. Duff. "The Spectrum of Tuberculosis in a New York City Men's Shelter Clinic (1982-1988)." *Chest* 97 (1990): 798-805.

15. Brudney and Dobkin, "Resurgent Tuberculosis in New York City."

16. "Tuberculosis, New York City." *City Health Information* 10, no. 2 (1991): 1-6.

17. E. Drucker, P. Alcabes, W. Bosworth, and B. Sckell. "Childhood Tuberculosis in the Bronx, New York." *Lancet* 343 (1994): 1482-85.

18. K. A. Sepkowitz, E. E. Telzak, S. Recalde, and D. Armstrong. "Trends in Susceptibility of Tuberculosis in New York City, 1987-1991." *Clinical Infectious Diseases* 18 (1994): 755-59.

19. T. R. Frieden, T. Sterling, A. Pablos-Mendez, J. O. Kilburn, G. M. Cauthen, and S. W. Dooley. "The Emergence of Drug-Resistant Tuberculosis in New York City." *New England Journal of Medicine* 328 (1993): 521-26.

20. A. B. Bloch, G. M. Cauthen, I. M. Onarato, et al. "Nationwide Survey of Resistant Tuberculosis in the United States." *Journal of the American Medical Association* 271 (1994): 665-71.

21. "Tuberculosis, New York City."

22. McAdam et al., "Spectrum of Tuberculosis in a New York City Men's Shelter Clinic"; E. Nardell, B. McInnis, B. Thomas, and S. Weidhaas. "Exogenous Reinfection with Tuberculosis in a Shelter for the Homeless." *New England Journal of Medicine* 315 (1986): 1570-75; A. Pablos-Mendez, M. C. Raviglione, B. Ruggero, and R. Ramox-Zuniga. "Drug-Resistant Tuberculosis among the Homeless in New York City." *New York State Journal of Medicine* 90 (1990): 351-55.

23. Author interview with W. El-Sadr, October 21, 1997.

24. H. Abeles, H. Feibes, E. Mandel, and J. A. Girard. "The Large City Prison—A Reservoir of Tuberculosis. Tuberculosis Control among Sentenced Male Prisoners in New York City." *American Review of Respiratory Disease* 10, no. 1 (1970): 706-9.

25. Centers for Disease Control. "Nosocomial Transmission of Multidrug-Resistant Tuberculosis among HIV-infected Persons—Florida and New York, 1988-1991." *Morbidity and Mortality Weekly Report* 40 (1991): 585-91; M. L. Pearson, J. A. Jereb, T. R. Frieden, et al. "Nosocomial Transmission of Multidrug-Resistant Mycobacterium Tuberculosis: A Risk to Patients and Health Workers." *Annals of Internal Medicine* 117 (1992): 191-96; S. E.

Valway, R. B. Greifinger, M. Papania, et al. "Multidrug-Resistant Tuberculosis in the New York State Prison System, 1990-1991." *Journal of Infectious Disease* 170 (1994): 151-56.

26. Centers for Disease Control. "Nosocomial Transmission of Multidrug-Resistant Tuberculosis."

27. Valway et al., "Multidrug-Resistant Tuberculosis in the New York State Prison System."

28. S. E. Valway, S. B. Richards, J. Kovacovich, R. B. Grelfinger, J. T.Crawford, and S. W. Dooley. "Outbreak of Multi-Drug-Resistant Tuberculosis in a New York State Prison, 1991." *American Journal of Epidemiology* 140, no. 2 (1994): 113-22; "Dealing with the TB Menace." *New York Post,* October 9, 1992, 28.

29. T. R. Frieden, L. F. Sherman, K. L. Maw, et al. "A Multi-Institutional Outbreak of Highly Drug-Resistant Tuberculosis." *Journal of the American Medical Association* 276 (1996): 1229-35.

30. T. R. Frieden, C. L. Woodley, J. T. Crawford, D. Lew, and S. M. Dooley. "The Molecular Epidemiology of Tuberculosis in New York City: The Importance of Nosocomial Transmission and Laboratory Error." *Tubercle and Lung Disease* 77 (1996): 407-13.

31. M. A. Fischl, G. L. Daikos, R. B. Uttamchandani, et al. "Clinical Presentation and Outcome of Patients with HIV Infection and Tuberculosis Caused by Multiple-Drug Resistant Bacilli." *Annals of Internal Medicine* 117 (1992): 184-90.

32. Frieden et al., "Emergence of Drug-Resistant Tuberculosis in New York City."

33. T. R. Frieden, P. I. Fujiwara, R. M. Washko, and M. A. Hamburg. "Tuberculosis in New York City—Turning the Tide." *New England Journal of Medicine* 333 (1995): 229-33.

34. *New Approach to a Resurging Crisis.* Report of the Task Force on Tuberculosis in New York, 1980. New York: Council of Lung Associations of New York, 1981.

35. *Tuberculosis in New York City, 1978.* New York: New York Lung Association, 1979.

36. K. E. Powell, E. D. Brown, and L. S. Farer. "Tuberculosis among Indochinese Refugees in the United States." *Journal of the American Medical Association* 249 (1983): 1455-60; Centers for Disease Control. "Tuberculosis in Philippine National World War II Veterans Immigrating to Hawaii, 1992-1993." *Morbidity and Mortality Weekly Report* 42 (1993): 656-63.

37. E. Bellin. "Failure of Tuberculosis Control: A Prescription for Change." *Journal of the American Medical Association* 271 (1994): 708-9.

38. *Report of the Task Force on Tuberculosis in New York City, 1968.* New York: New York Lung Association, 1968.

39. *Tuberculosis in New York City, 1970.* New York: New York Lung Association, 1971.

40. *Tuberculosis in New York City, 1977.* New York Lung Association, 1978.

41. Brudney and Dobkin, "A Tale of Two Cities."

42. K. Brudney. "Homelessness and TB: A Study in Failure." *Journal of Law, Medicine, and Ethics* 21, nos. 3-4 (1993): 360-67.

43. "Tuberculosis." *City Health Information* 15, no. 4 (1996): 12-13.

44. Brudney and Dobkin, "Resurgent Tuberculosis in New York City."
45. *Tuberculosis in New York City, 1984-1985;* P. I. Fujiwara, C. Larkin, and T. R. Frieden. "Directly Observed Therapy in New York City." *Clinics in Chest Medicine* 18, no. 1 (1997): 135-48.
46. Brudney and Dobkin, "Resurgent Tuberculosis in New York City."
47. *Tuberculosis in New York City, 1988.* New York: New York City Department of Health, 1990.
48. K. D. Davis, D. Rowland, K. S. Altman, K. S. Collins, and C. Morris. "Health Insurance: The Size and Shape of the Problem." *Inquiry* 32 (summer 1995): 196-203.
49. G. Claxton. *Reform of the Individual Health Insurance Market.* New York: The Commonwealth Fund, 1996.
50. Employee Benefit Research Institute. *Sources of Health Insurance and Characteristics of the Uninsured: Analysis of March 1991 Current Population Survey.* Washington, DC: EBRI, 1992.
51. Author interview with G. Cairns, March 23, 1998.
52. J. Feder, J. Hadley, and R. Mullner. "Falling through the Cracks: Poverty, Insurance Coverage, and Hospitals' Care to the Poor 1980 and 1982." In: S. J. Robers, A. M. Rousseau, S. W. Nesbitt, and J. Griggs, eds. *Hospitals and the Uninsured Poor: Based on the Proceedings of a United Hospital Fund Conference.* New York: United Hospitals Fund of New York, 1985.
53. General Accounting Office. *Health Insurance: An Overview of the Working Uninsured.* Washington, DC: GAO, 1989.
54. General Accounting Office. *Private Health Insurance: Problems Caused by a Segmented Market.* Washington, DC: GAO, 1991.
55. *Medicaid Source Book: Background Data and Analysis.* Washington, DC: Government Printing Office, 1988.
56. K. Davis and D. Rowland. "Financing Health Care for the Poor." In: E. Ginzberg, ed., *Health Services Research: Key to Health Policy.* Cambridge, MA: Harvard University Press, 1991.
57. Brudney and Dobkin, "Resurgent Tuberculosis in New York City"; E. Rosenthal. "Health Problems of Inner City Poor Reach Crisis Point." *New York Times,* December 24, 1990: A1, A9; D. Martin. "Economic Ills: Poor Are Sicker, Clinic Is Poorer." *New York Times,* March 6, 1991: B1; J. M. Colwill. "Where Have All the Primary Care Applicants Gone?" *New England Journal of Medicine* 326 (1992): 387-93.
58. Cairns interview.
59. Ibid.
60. K. Davies and D. Rowland. "Uninsured and Underserved: Inequities in Health Care in the United States." *Milbank Memorial Fund Quarterly* 61 (1983): 149-76; J. Weissman and A. M. Epstein. "Case Mix and Resource Utilization by Uninsured Hospital Patients in the Boston Metropolitan Area." *Journal of the American Medical Association* 261 (1991): 3572-76; P. A. Braveman, S. Egerter, T. Bennett, and J. Showstack. "Differences in Hospital Resource Allocation among Sick Newborns According to Insurance Coverage." *Journal of the American Medical Association* 266 (1991): 3300-8.
61. Employee Benefit Research Institute, *Sources of Health Insurance;* G. A. Kaplan, E. R. Pamuk, J. W. Lynch, R. D. Cohen, and J. L. Balfour.

"Inequality in Income and Mortality in the United States: Analysis of Mortality and Potential Pathways." *British Medical Journal* 312 (1996): 999-1003.

62. J. Hadley, E. P. Steinberg, and J. Feder. "Comparison of Uninsured and Privately Insured Hospital Patients: Conditions on Admission, Resource Use, and Outcome." *Journal of the American Medical Association* 265 (1991): 374-79.

63. G. Anderson. "In Search of Value: An International Comparison of Cost, Access, and Outcomes." *Health Affairs* 16, no. 6 (1997): 163-71; M. Schlesinger and K. Kronebsch. "The Failure of Prenatal Care Policy for the Poor." *Health Affairs* 9 (1990): 91-111.

64. C. J. Syverson, W. Chavkin, H. K. Atrash, R. W. Rochat, E. S. Sharp, and G. E. King. "Pregnancy-related Mortality in New York, 1980 to 1984: Causes of Death and Associated Risk Factors." *American Journal of Obstetrics and Gynecology* 164 (1991): 603-8.

65. C. McCord and H. P. Freeman. "Excess Mortality in Harlem." *New England Journal of Medicine* 322 (1990): 173-77.

66. Anderson, "In Search of Value."

67. U. Reinhardt. "Paying the Doctor: Lessons from Home and Abroad." Annual Conference of the New York Academy of Medicine. New York, 1987.

68. M. Michael. "Slouching toward Chaos: American Health Policy and the Homeless." In: P. W. Brickner, L. K. Scharer, B. A. Conanan, M. Savarese, and B. C. Scanlan, eds. *Under the Safety Net: The Health and Social Welfare of the Homeless in the United States.* New York: W. W. Norton, 1992.

69. Brudney, "Homelessness and TB."

70. Brudney and Dobkin, "Resurgent Tuberculosis in New York City"; Nardell et al., "Exogenous Reinfection with Tuberculosis."

71. *1990 Census of the U.S. Population.* Washington, DC: U.S. Department of Commerce, Bureau of the Census, 1992.

72. D. Wallace. "Roots of Increased Health Care Inequality in New York." *Social Science and Medicine* 31, no. 11 (1990): 1219-27.

73. R. Wallace. "Contagion and Incubation in New York City Structural Fires, 1964-76." *Human Ecology* 6, no. 4 (1978): 423-33; R. Wallace. "Fire Service Productivity and the New York City Fire Crisis: 1968-1979." *Human Ecology* 9, no. 4 (1981): 433-64.

74. R. Wallace and D. Wallace. "Origins of Public Health Collapse in New York City: The Dynamics of Planned Shrinkage, Contagious Urban Decay and Social Disintegration." *Bulletin of the New York Academy of Medicine* 66, no. 5 (1990): 391-434.

75. R. Schaffer and N. Smith. "The Gentrification of Harlem?" *Annals of the Association of American Geographers* 76 (1986): 347-65.

76. OMB Watch, 1990; Committee on Health Care for Homeless People, Institute of Medicine. *Homelessness, Health, and Human Needs.* Washington, DC: National Academy Press, 1988; M. B. Katz. *In the Shadow of the Poorhouse: A Social History of Welfare in America.* New York: Basic Books, 1986; M. B. Katz. *The Undeserving Poor: From the War on Poverty to the War on Welfare.* New York: Pantheon Books, 1989; C. Hartman. "Housing Policies under the Reagan Administration." In: R. G. Bratt, C. Hartman, and

A. Meyerson, eds. *Critical Perspectives on Housing*. Philadelphia: Temple University Press, 1986.

77. Hartman, "Housing Polices under the Reagan Administration."
78. M. Stegman. *Housing and vacancy report: New York City, 1987*. New York: New York City Department of Housing Preservation and Development, 1988.
79. J. Hughes and G. Sternlieb. *Rutgers Regional Report: Volume 1: Job, Income, Population and Housing Baselines*. New Brunswick, NJ: Rutgers University, 1989.
80. J. D. Kasarda. "Urban Change and Minority Opportunities." In: P. Peterson, ed., *The New Urban Reality*. Washington, DC: The Brookings Institution, 1985.
81. Wallace, "Roots of Increased Health Care Inequality in New York"; Wallace and Wallace, "Origins of Public Health Collapse in New York City."
82. Brickner et al., *Under the Safety Net;* F. Barringer. "Federal Count of Homeless Is Far Below Other Figures," *New York Times,* April 12, 1991: A14; P. W. Brickner, L. K. Sharer, B. Conanan , A. Elvy, and M. Savarese, eds. *Health Care of Homeless People*. New York: Springer, 1985; E. F. Torrey. "Nowhere to Go: The Tragic Odyssey of the Homeless Mentally Ill." *American Journal of Psychiatry* 141, no. 4 (1984): 975-78.
83. C. W. Dugger. "Study Says Shelter Turnover Hides Scope of Homelessness." *New York Times,* November 16, 1993: Al.
84. Brickner et al., *Under the Safety Net*.
85. *The Second Wave: The Looming Homeless Crisis in the Post-Entitlement Era*. New York: Coalition for the Homeless, 1996.
86. J. Q. La Fond and M. L. Durham. *Back to the Asylum: The Future of Mental Health Law and Policy in the United States*. New York: Oxford University Press, 1992.
87. Ibid.
88. M. R. Burt and B. E. Cohen. *America's Homeless: Numbers, Characteristics, and Programs That Serve Them*. Washington, DC: Urban University Press, 1989; P. H. Rossi. *Down and Out in America: The Origins of Homelessness*. Chicago: University of Chicago Press, 1989.
89. *Statistical Abstract of the United States*. Washington, DC: U.S. Department of Commerce, Bureau of the Census, 1988.
90. M. Harloe, P. Marcuse, and N. Smith. "Housing for People, Housing for Profits." In: S. S. Fainstein, I. Gordon, and M. Harloe, eds. *Divided Cities: New York & London in the Contemporary World*. Oxford: Blackwell, 1992.
91. J. Austin and A. D. McVey. *The 1989 NCCD Prison Population Forecast: The Impact of the War on Drugs*. San Francisco: The National Council on Crime and Delinquency, 1989; *Federal Sentencing in Transition, 1986-1990*. Washington, DC: Department of Justice, 1992.
92. Washington, DC: Bureau of Justice Statistics, U.S. Department of Justice, Office of Justice Programs, 1992.
93. *Annual Report*. Albany: New York State Department of Corrections, 1989.
94. T. J. Flanagan and K. Maguire, eds. *Sourcebook of Criminal Justice Statistics, 1989*. Washington, DC: U.S. Department of Justice, Bureau of Justice Statistics, 1990; "National Household Survey on Drug Abuse." National

Institute on Drug Abuse (NIDA), 1990.

95. T. Duster. "Pattern, Purpose, and Race in the Drug War: The Crisis of Credibility in Criminal Justice." In: C. Reinarman and H. G. Levine, eds., *Crack in America: Demon Drugs and Social Justice.* Berkeley: University of California Press, 1997.

96. Ibid.

97. "Young Black Men and the Criminal Justice System: A Growing National Problem." The Sentencing Project, 1990.

98. *Imprisoned Generation.* New York: Correctional Association of New York and the New York State Coalition for Criminal Justice, 1990.

99. I. Glasser and L. Siegel, "'When Constitutional Rights Seem Too Extravagant to Endure': The Crack Scare's Impact on Civil Rights and Liberties." In: C. Reinarman and H. G. Levine, eds., *Crack in America: Demon Drugs and Social Justice.* Berkeley, University of California Press, 19997.

100. Section 21 U.S.C. 841(a).

101. D. C. Des Jarlais, S. R. Friedman, D. Novick, et al. "HIV-1 Infection among Intravenous Drug Users in Manhattan, New York City, from 1977 through 1987." *Journal of the American Medical Association* 261 (1989): 1008-12; D.C. Des Jarlais, M. Marmor, D. Paone, et al. "HIV Incidence among Injecting Drug Users in New York City Syringe-Exchange Programmes." *Lancet* 348 (1996): 987-91.

102. R. Bayer. *Private Acts, Social Consequences: AIDS and the Politics of Public Health.* New York City: The Free Press, 1989.

103. A. Waterston. "Anthropological Research and the Politics of HIV Prevention: Towards a Critique of Policy and Priorities in the Age of AIDS." *Social Science and Medicine* 44 (1997): 1381-91.

104. J.-P. C. Grund, L. S. Stem, C. D. Kaplan, N. F. P. Adriaans, and E. Drucker. "Drug use Contexts and HIV Consequences: The Effect of Drug Policy on Patterns of Everyday Drug Use in Rotterdam and the Bronx." *British Journal of Addiction* 87 (1992): 381-92.

105. L. M. Kochems, D. Paone, D. C. Des Jarlais, I. Ness, J. Clark, and S. R. Friedman. "The Transition from Underground to Legal Syringe Exchange: The New York City Experience." *AIDS Education and Prevention* 8 (1996): 471-89.

106. W. N. Elwood, M. L. Williams, D. C. Bell, and A. J. Richard. "Powerlessness and HIV Prevention among People Who Trade Sex for Drug ('Strawberries')." *AIDS Care* 9 (1997): 273-84.

107. Ibid.; S. Zierler and N. Krieger. "Reframing Women's Risk: Social Inequalities and HIV Infection." *Annual Review of Public Health* 18 (1997): 401-36; J. A. Inciardi. "Crack, Crack House Sex, and HIV Risk." *Archives of Sexual Behavior* 24 (1995): 249-69; A. Pivnick, A. Jacobson, E. Eric, L. Doll, and E. Drucker. "AIDS, HIV Infection, and Illicit Drug Use within Inner-City Families and Social Networks." *American Journal of Public Health* 84 (1994): 271-74.

108. P. M. Brien and A. J. Beck. *HIV in Prisons 1994.* Washington, DC: Bureau of Justice Statistics, 1996.

109. N. Mahon. "New York Inmates' HIV Risk Behaviours: The Implications for Prevention Policy and Programs." *American Journal of Public Health* 86

(1996): 1211-15.

110. Ibid.; A. J. Beck, D. K. Gilliard, L. Greenfeld, et al. *Survey of State Prison Inmates, 1991.* Washington, DC: National Institute of Justice, 1993; S. R. Donziger, ed. *The Real War on Crime.* New York: Harper, 1996; R. C. Horsburgh, J. Q. Jarvis, T. McArthur, R. N. Ignacio, and P. Stock. "Seroconversion to Human Immunodeficiency Virus in Prison Inmates." *American Journal of Public Health* 80 (1990): 209-10; R. C. Mutter, R. M. Grimes, and D. Labarthe. "Evidence of Intraprison Spread of HIV Infection." *Archives of Internal Medicine* 154 (1994): 793-95.

111. Bayer, *Private Acts, Social Consequences.*

112. S. G. Stolberg. "Clinton Decides Not to Finance Needle Program." *New York Times,* April 21, 1998: AI, A18.

113. S. A. Mednick, W. F. Gabrielli, and B. Hutchings. "Genetic Influences in Criminal Convictions: Evidence from an Adoption Cohort." *Science,* May 25, 1984: 891-94; H. Yoshikawa. "Prevention as Cumulative Protection: Effects of Early Family Support and Education on Chronic Delinquency and Its Risks." *Psychological Bulletin* 115, no. 1 (1994): 28-54.

114. H. Yoshikawa. "Long-term Effects of Early Childhood Programs on Social Outcomes and Delinquency." *The Future of Children* 5, no. 3 (winter 1995): 51-75.

115. J. W. C. Johnstone. "Social Class, Social Areas and Delinquency." *Sociology and Social Research* 63 (1978): 49-72.

116. J. Fishkin. *Justice, Equal Opportunity and the Family.* New Haven, CT: Yale University Press, 1983.

117. A. Hirschman and M. Rothschild. "The Changing Tolerance for Income Inequality in the Course of Economic Development." *Quarterly Journal of Economics* 87 (1973): 546.

118. D. R. Schaffer. *Social and Personality Development,* 3rd ed. Pacific Grove, CA: Brooks/Cole Publishing Company, 1994; D. P. McAdams. *The Person: An Introduction to Personality Psychology.* London: Harcourt Brace Jovanovich, 1990.

119. V. E. Frankl. *Man's Search for Meaning,* 4th ed. Boston: Beacon Press, 1992.

120. H. S. Becker. *Outsiders: Studies in the Sociology of Deviance.* Glencoe, IL: Free Press of Glencoe, 1963.

121. L. J. D. Wacquant and W. J. Wison. "The Cost of Racial and Class Exclusion in the Inner City." In: W. J. Wilson, ed., *The Ghetto Underclass.* Newbury Park, CA: Sage Publications, 1993: 25-42.

122. Author interview with M. T. Fullilove, March 24, 1998.

123. I. Wilkerson. "Crack Means Power, and Death, to Soldiers in Street Wars." *New York Times,* December 13, 1994.

124. Wallace, "Roots of Increased Health Care Inequality"; Wallace and Wallace, "Origins of Public Health Collapse in New York City."

125. M. Hout. "The Politics of Mobility." In: A. C. Kerckhoff, ed., *Generations and the Lifecourse.* Boulder, CO: Westview Press, 1995.

126. M. Hout. "Expanding Universalism, Less Structural Mobility: The American Occupational Structure in the 1980s." *American Journal of Sociology* 93 (1988): 1358-1400.

127. F. Levy. "Incomes and Income Inequality." In: R. Farley, ed., *State of the*

Union: America in the 1990s. New York: Russell Sage Foundation, 1995.

128. W. J. Wilson. *The Truly Disadvantaged: The Inner City, the Underclass, and Public Policy.* Chicago: University of Chicago Press, 1987.

129. S. Bowles and H. Gintis. *Schooling in Capitalist America: Education and the Contradictions of Economic Life.* New York: Basic Books, 1976.

130. Kasarda, "Urban Change and Minority Opportunities."

131. Katz, *The Undeserving Poor.*

132. J. D. Kasarda. "Urban Industrial Transition and the Underclass." In: W. J. Wilson, ed., *The Ghetto Underclass.* Newbury Park, CA: Sage Publications, 1993.

133. T. Bailey. "Black Employment Opportunities." In: C. Brecher and R. D. Horton, eds., *Setting Municipal Priorities, 1990.* New York: New York University Press, 1989.

134. P. Townsend. *Poverty in the United Kingdom: A Survey of Household Resources and Standards of Living.* Berkeley: University of California Press, 1979.

135. Wilson, *The Truly Disadvantaged.*

136. M. Harrington. *The New American Poverty.* New York: Holt, Rinehart, and Winston, 1984; L. Beeghley. "Illusion and Reality in the Measurement of Poverty." *Social Problems* 31 (1984): 335.

137. R. Sidel. *Women and Children Last: The Plight of Poor Women in Affluent America,* rev. ed. New York City: Penguin Books, 1992; V. W. Sidel. "The Health of Poor and Minority People in the Inner City." *New York State Journal of Medicine* 91 (1991): 180-82.

138. Sidel, *Women and Children Last.*

139. R. B. Mincy and S. J. Wiener. *The Underclass in the 1980s: Changing Concept, Constant Reality.* Washington, DC: Urban Institute, 1993.

140. P. A. Jargowsky and M. J. Bane. "Ghetto Poverty in the United States, 1970-1980." In: C. Jencks and P. E. Peterson, eds., *The Urban Underclass.* Washington, DC: The Brookings Institution, 1991.

141. Wilson, *The Truly Disadvantaged;* D. T. Ellwood. *Poor Support: Poverty in the American Family.* New York: Basic Books, 1988.

142. Jargowsky and Bane, "Ghetto Poverty in the United States."

143. Katz, *The Undeserving Poor.*

144. U.S. Department of Commerce, Bureau of the Census.

145. P. Gottschalk P and T. M. Smeeding. "Cross-national Comparisons of Earnings and Income Inequality." *Journal of Economic Literature* 35 (1997): 633-87.

146. D. U. Himmelstein and S. Woolhandler. *The National Health Program Chartbook,* vol 24. Cambridge: Center for National Health Program Studies, 1992.

147. C. S. Fischer, M. Hout, M. S. Jankowski, S. R. Lucas, A. Swidler, and K. Voss. *Inequality by Design: Cracking the Bell Curve Myth.* Princeton, NJ: Princeton University Press, 1996.

148. Ibid.; G. A. Crystal. *In Search of Excess: The Overcompensation of American Executives.* New York: W. W. Norton, 1991.

149. K. Larin and E. McNichol. *The Long-Term Trend: The Late 1970s to the Mid-1990s. Pulling Apart: A State-by-State Analysis of Income Trends.* Washington, DC: Center on Budget and Policy Priorities, 1997.

150. Fischer et al., *Inequality by Design.*
151. J. L. Palmer and I. V. Sawhill, eds. *The Reagan Experiment.* Washington, DC: Urban Institute Press, 1982.

CHAPTER 4

1. S. C. Joseph. "New York City, Tuberculosis, and the Public Health Infrastructure." *Journal of Law, Medicine, and Ethics* 21, nos. 3-4 (1993): 372-75.
2. Author interview with W. El-Sadr, October 21, 1997.
3. Centers for Disease Control. "Strategic Plan for the Elimination of Tuberculosis in the United States." *Morbidity and Mortality Weekly Report* (1989): 38.
4. R. J. Coker. "Uncertainty, Civil Liberties, Coercion, and Public Health." *British Medical Journal* 318 (1999): 1434-35.
5. C. H. Foreman Jr. *Plagues, Products & Politics: Emergent Public Health Hazards and National Policymaking.* Washington, DC: The Brookings Institution, 1994.
6. Author interview with T. R. Frieden, June 29, 1998.
7. Foreman, *Plagues, Products & Politics.*
8. A. V. Bollinger. "TB Timebomb. Homeless Contaminate Public Areas in City." *New York Post,* October 16, 1990: 4, 18.
9. A. V. Bollinger. "Highly Contagious Tuberculosis Close to Epidemic Level in the City." *New York Post,* October 17, 1990: 1.
10. L. K. Altman. "Deadly Strain of Tuberculosis Is Spreading Fast, U.S. Finds." *New York Times,* January 24, 1992: Al, B6.
11. L. K. Altman. "For Most, Risk of Contracting Tuberculosis Is Seen as Small." *New York Times,* January 25, 1992: Al, B9.
12. K. Chowder. "TB: The Disease That Rose from Its Grave." *Smithsonian* (November 1992): 180-96.
13. "Safeguarding the City against TB." *New York Post,* February 25, 1992:20.
14. "Can Society Protect Itself?" *New York Post,* September 5, 1992: 12.
15. "Dealing with the TB Menace." *New York Post,* October 9, 1992: 28.
16. M. Specter. "Neglected for Years, TB Is Back with Strains That Are Deadlier." *New York Times,* October 11, 1992: 1, 44; E. Rosenthal. "Doctors and Patients Are Pushed to Their Limits by Grim New TB." *New York Times,* October 12, 1992: Al, B2; E. Rosenthal. "TB, Easily Transmitted, Adds a Peril to Medicine." *New York Times,* October 13, 1992: A1, B1; M. Specter. "TB Carriers See Clash of Liberty and Health." *New York Times,* October 14, 1992: Al, B4; L. K. Altman. "Stymied by Resurgence of TB, Doctors Reconsider a Decades-old Vaccine. *New York Times,* October 15, 1992: 134.
17. Specter, "Neglected for Years, TB Is Back."
18. Ibid.
19. Rosenthal, "TB, Easily Transmitted, Adds a Peril to Medicine."
20. New York City. *TB Control Interactive Strategic Planning.* New York: The Fund for the City of New York, 1992.
21. D. Garey and L. R. Holt. *The People's Plague: Tuberculosis in America.* Florentine Films, 1995.
22. *Tuberculosis in New York City, 1984-1985.* New York City Department of Health: 1987.

23. Centers for Disease Control. "Review of Tuberculosis Prevention and Control Activities in New York City." *Morbidity and Mortality Weekly Report* (November 1987).

24. Joseph, "New York City, Tuberculosis, and the Public Health Infrastructure."

25. Expert Advisory Committee on Tuberculosis. *Report to the Commissioner.* New York: New York City Department of Health, 1988.

26. Joseph, "New York City, Tuberculosis, and the Public Health Infrastructure."

27. M. S. Dorsinville. "Case Management of Tuberculosis in New York City." *International Journal of Tuberculosis and Lung Disease* 2, no. 9 (1998): S46-S52; author interview with Frieden.

28. New York Academy of Medicine Committee on Single Disease Institutions for Tuberculosis. "Recommendations on the Facilities Needed to Care for Patients with Tuberculosis. In: D. J. Rothman, ed., *The Tuberculosis Revival: Individual Rights and Societal Obligations in a Time of AIDS.* New York: United Hospital Fund, 1992.

29. D. J. Rothman. "The Single Disease Hospital: Why Tuberculosis Justifies a Departure that AIDS Does Not. *Journal of Law, Medicine, and Ethics* 21, nos. 3-4 (1993): 296-302.

30. K. Brudney and J. Dobkin. "A Tale of Two Cities: Tuberculosis Control in Managua and New York City." *Seminars in Respiratory Infections* 6 (1991): 261-72.

31. Rothman, "Single Disease Hospital."

32. New York Academy of Medicine Committee, "Recommendations on the Facilities. Needed to Care for Patients with Tuberculosis.

33. Working Group on Tuberculosis and HIV. "Tuberculosis in the 1990s: Ethical, Legal, and Public Policy Issues in Screening, Treatment, and the Protection of Those in Congregate Facilities." In: N. N. Dubler, R. Bayer, S. Landesman, and A. White, eds. *The Tuberculosis Revival: Individual Rights and Societal Obligations in a Time of AIDS.* New York: United Hospital Fund, 1992.

34. Ibid.

35. Ibid.

36. Frieden interview.

37. *Tuberculosis (TB) Blueprint: Goals and Objectives (draft).* New York: Commissioner's Office, New York City Department of Health, 1992.

38. Ibid.

39. Dorsinville, "Case Management of Tuberculosis"; T. R. Frieden, P. I. Fujiwara, R. M. Washko, and M. A. Hamburg. "Tuberculosis in New York City—Turning the Tide." *New England Journal of Medicine* 333 (1995): 229-33.

40. Dorsinville, "Case Management of Tuberculosis."

41. Frieden et al., "Tuberculosis in New York City."

42. Ibid.; Memorandum from Cesar A. Perales to Mayor David N. Dinkins. Update on tuberculosis (TB) Control Activities. New York: Office of the Mayor, 1993.

43. Centers for Disease Control. "Guidelines for Preventing the Transmission of Mycobacterium tuberculosis in Health-Care Facilities, 1994." *Morbidity and Mortality Weekly Report* (1994) (No. RR-13).

44. M. L. Pearson, J. A. Jereb, T. R. Frieden, et al. "Nosocomial Transmission of Multidrug-Resistant Mycobacterium tuberculosis: A Risk to Patients and Health Workers." *Annals of Internal Medicine* 117 (1992): 191-96; B. Nivin, P. Nicholas, M. Gayer, T. R. Frieden, and P. I. Fujiwara. "A Continuing Outbreak of Multidrug-Resistant Tuberculosis, with Transmission in a Hospital Nursery." *Clinical Infectious Diseases* 26, no. 2 (1998): 303-7.

45. Frieden et al., "Tuberculosis in New York City"; *Tuberculosis (TB) Blueprint.*

46. D. Broderick. "Judge: Add TB Ward to Rikers." *New York Post,* January 25, 1992: 8.

47. S. E. Valway, S. B. Richards, J. Kovacovich, R. B. Greifinger, J. T. Crawford, and S. W. Dooley. "Outbreak of Multi-Drug-Resistant Tuberculosis in a New York State Prison, 1991." *American Journal of Epidemiology* 140, no. 2 (1994): 113-22.

48. Memorandum from Perales to Dinkins.

49. T. R. Frieden, L. F. Sherman, K. L. Maw, et al. "A Multi-Institutional Outbreak of Highly Drug-Resistant Tuberculosis." *Journal of the American Medical Association* 276 (1996): 1229-35; L. C. Klopf. "Tuberculosis Control in the New York State Department of Corrections Services: A Case Management Approach." *American Journal of Infection Control* 25, no. 5 (1998): 534-4-7.

50. New York City TB Control Interactive Strategic Planning.

51. R. B. Greifinger. "Tuberculosis behind Bars." In: N. N. Dubler, R. Bayer, S. Landesman, and A. White, eds. *The Tuberculosis Revival: Individual Rights and Societal Obligations in a Time of AIDS.* New York: United Hospital Fund, 1992.

52. Dorsinville, "Case Management of Tuberculosis"; "Tuberculosis." *City Health Information* 15, no. 4 (1996): 12-13.

53. Memorandum from Perales to Dinkins.

54. Advisory Council for the Elimination of Tuberculosis. "Initial Therapy for Tuberculosis in the Era of Multidrug Resistance: Recommendations of the Advisory Council for the Elimination of Tuberculosis." *Morbidity and Mortality Weekly Report* 42 (1993) (no. RR/7).

55. R. Bayer and D. Wilkinson. "Directly Observed Therapy for Tuberculosis: History of an Idea." *Lancet* 345 (1995): 1545.

56. P. I. Fujiwara, C. Larkin, and T. R. Frieden. "Directly Observed Therapy in New York City." *Clinics in Chest Medicine* 8, no. 1 (1997): 135-48.

57. Ibid.

58. Specter, "TB Carriers See Clash of Liberty and Health."

59. Tuberculosis (TB) Blueprint.

60. Frieden interview; M. R. Gasner, personal communication, 1998; M. R. Gasner, K. L. Maw, G. E. Feldman, P. I. Fujiwara, and T. R. Frieden. "The Use of Legal Action in New York City to Ensure Treatment of Tuberculosis." *New England Journal of Medicine* 340 (1998): 359-66.

61. Author interview with L. Nathan, March 13, 1998.

62. Author interview with N. Schluger, October 15, 1997.

63. Author interview with S. S. Munsiff, October 17, 1997; Author interview with M. Barnes, December 9, 1997.

64. Barnes interview.

65. El-Sadr interview.

66. "Notice of Adoption of an Amendment to Section 11.47 of the New York City Health Code." New York: Department of Health, Board of Health, 1993.

67. New York City, N.Y., Health Code 11.55 (1993).

68. C. A. Ball and M. Barnes. "Public Health and Individual Rights: Tuberculosis Control and Detention Procedures in New York City." *Yale Law and Policy Review* 12, no. 1 (1994): 38-67.

69. "Minutes of Meeting." New York: New York City Board of Health, 1992.

70. Ibid.

71. Request to Amend Section 11.47 Health Code. From Kenneth Ong, Deputy Commissioner of Disease Intervention to Margaret Hamburg, Commissioner of Health, New York City, October 6, 1992.

72. Ibid.

73. Proposed Amendments to Section 11.47 of New York City Health Code.

74. New York Academy of Medicine Committee on Single Disease Institutions for Tuberculosis, "Recommendations."

75. New York City Tuberculosis Working Group. "Developing a System for Tuberculosis Prevention and Care in New York City." In: N. N. Dubler, R. Bayer, S. Landesman, and A. White, eds. *The Tuberculosis Revival: Individual Rights and Societal Obligations in a Time of AIDS*. New York City: United Hospitals Fund, 1992.

76. Ibid.

77. Public hearing of the proposed amendment to Section 11.47 of the New York City Health Code. New York City: Department of Health, Board of Health, 1992.

78. New York City Tuberculosis Working Group, "Developing a System."

79. Rothman, "Single Disease Hospital"; New York Tuberculosis Working Group. Response to Tom Frieden at Public Meeting, New York City.

80. Public hearing of proposed amendment.

81. Ibid.; Rosenthal, "TB, Easily Transmitted, Adds a Peril."

82. Public hearing to proposed amendment.

83. Ibid.

84. Response to public comments concerning proposed amendments to Section 11.47 of Health Code. To: Hamburg, M; From: Henning, K. New York: Department of Health, 1993.

85. Centers for Disease Control. "Tuberculosis Control Laws—United States, 1993." *Morbidity and Mortality Weekly Report* 42 (1993) (no. RR15).

86. *City v. Antoinette R.*, 165 Misc. 2d 1014, 630 N.Y.S.2d 1008 (Sup. 1995).

87. Court Hearing, September 13, 1998, Goldwater Memorial Hospital.

88. *O'Connor v. Donaldson*, 422 U.S. 563, 575 (1975).

89. E. Sumartojo. "When Tuberculosis Treatment Fails: A Social Behavioural Account of Patient Adherence." *American Review of Respiratory Disease* 147 (1993): 1311-20.

90. *Addington v. Texas* 441 U.S. 418, 427 (1979).

91. New York City Tuberculosis Working Group, "Developing a System for Tuberculosis Prevention"; L. O. Gostin. "Controlling the Resurgent Tuberculosis Epidemic: A 50-State Survey of TB Statutes and Proposals for

Reform." *Journal of the American Medical Association* 269, no. 2 (1993): 255-61.

92. Americans with Disabilities Act of 1990, 42 USC.

93. L. O. Gostin. "The Resurgent Tuberculosis Epidemic in the Era of AIDS: Reflections on Public Health, Law, and Society." *Maryland Law Review* 54, no. 1 (1995): 131.

94. Americans with Disabilities Act of 1990, 42 USC; L. O. Gostin. "Public Health Powers: The Imminence of Radical Change." In: Conference Proceedings, *The Dual Epidemics of Tuberculosis and AIDS: Health Care Policy, professional Practice, Law and Ethics*. New York City, (December 4-5, 1992): 268-90.

95. Ball and Barnes, "Public Health and Individual Rights."

96. *School Board of Nassau County, Fl. v. Arline,* 480 U.S. 273, 288 (1987).

97. Ibid.

98. *Bragdon v. Abbott,* No. 97-156 (1998).

99. Americans with Disabilities Act.

100. *School Board of Nassau County, Fl. v. Arline.*

101. Gostin, "Conference Proceedings."

102. Gostin, "Resurgent Tuberculosis Epidemic."

103. Ball and Barnes, "Public Health and Individual Rights."

104. A. Alpers, T. Oscherwitz, and B. Lo. *Conference Proceedings: Detaining Nonadherent Tuberculosis Patients Until Cure: A 50-State Legal Survey. Policy and Legal Dilemmas Regarding Refractory Tuberculosis Patients.* Francis J. Curry National Tuberculosis Center: University of California, San Francisco, 1996.

105. Gostin, "Resurgent Tuberculosis Epidemic."

106. Public hearing of proposed amendment.

CHAPTER 5

1. T. R. Frieden, P. I. Fujiwara, R. M. Washko, and M. A. Hamburg. "Tuberculosis in New York City—Turning the Tide." *New England Journal of Medicine* 333 (1995): 229-33.

2. "Information Summary." New York: Bureau of Tuberculosis Control, New York City Department of Health, 1996; "Information Summary." New York: Bureau of Tuberculosis Control, New York City Department of Health, 1997.

3. "Information Summary 1997."

4. "Information Summary 1997"; *Tuberculosis in New York City, 1991.* New York: Bureau of Tuberculosis Control, Department of Health, 1991.

5. *Tuberculosis in New York City, 1992.* New York: Bureau of Tuberculosis Control, New York City Department of Health, 1992; "Information Summary." New York: Bureau of Tuberculosis Control, New York City Department of Health, 1995.

6. Frieden et al., "Tuberculosis in New York City."

7. N. J. Binkin, P. L. F. Zuber, C. D. Wells, M. A. Tipple, and K. G. Castro. "Overseas Screening for Tuberculosis in Immigrants and Refugees to the United States: Current Status." *Clinical Infectious Diseases* 23 (1996): 1226-32.

8. "Information Summary 1997."

9. L. C. Klopf. "Tuberculosis Control in the New York State Department of Corrections Services: A Case Management Approach." *American Journal of Infection Control* 26, no. 5 (1998): 534-5-7.

10. "Tuberculosis." *City Health Information* (CHI) 15, no. 4 (1996): 12-13; M. S. Dorsinville. "Case Management of Tuberculosis in New York City." *International Journal of Tuberculosis and Lung Disease* 2, no. 9 (1998):S 46-S52.

11. "Information Summary 1997."

12. Ibid.

13. M. Moore, I. M. Onorato, E. McCray, and K. G. Castro. "Trends in Drug-Resistant Tuberculosis in the United States, 1993-1996." *Journal of the American Medical Association* 278 (1997): 833-37.

14. Ibid.

15. P. I. Fujiwara, S. V. Cook, C. M. Rutherford, et al. "A Continuing Survey of Drug-Resistant Tuberculosis, New York City, April 1994." *Archives of Internal Medicine* 157 (1997): 531-36.

16. M. R. Gasner, K. L. Maw, G. E. Feldman, P. I. Fujiwara, and T. R. Frieden. "The Use of Legal Action in New York City to Ensure Treatment of Tuberculosis." *New England Journal of Medicine* 340 (1998): 359-66.

17. Ibid.

18. Author interview with L. Nathan, March 13, 1998.

19. Author interview with W. El-Sadr, October 21, 1997.

20. K. Brudney and J. Dobkin. "Resurgent Tuberculosis in New York City: Human Immunodeficiency Virus, Homelessness and the Decline of Tuberculosis Control Programmes." *American Review of Respiratory Disease* 144 (1991): 745-49.

21. W. El-Sadr, F. Medard, and M. Dickerson. "The Harlem Family Model: A Unique Approach to the Treatment of Tuberculosis." *Journal of Public Health Management and Practice* 1, no. 4 (1995): 48-51.

22. Author interview with L. A. Moed, January 22, 1998.

23. *City v. Cheryl Lee.* Supreme Court of the State of New York, County of Kings, 1993.

24. Centers for Disease Control. "Tuberculosis Control Laws—United States, 1993." *Morbidity and Mortality Weekly Report* 42, no. RR-15 (1993): 1-28.

25. A. Alpers, T. Oscherwitz, and B. Lo. Conference Proceedings: Detaining Nonadherent Tuberculosis Patients until Cure: A 50-state Legal Survey. Policy and Legal Dilemmas Regarding Refractory Tuberculosis Patients. Francis J. Curry National Tuberculosis Center: University of California, San Francisco, 1996; Massachusetts General Law, Ch. 111, Sections 94, A-H; Maryland State Law, An. Code 1957, 8-325.

26. T. Oscherwitz, J. P. Tulsky, S. Roger, et al. "Detention of Persistently Nonadherent Patient with Tuberculosis." *Journal of the American Medical Association* 278 (1997): 843-46.

27. Author interview with R. Chaisson, November 11, 1997; W. J. Burman, D. L. Cohn, C. A. Rietmetjer, F. N. Judson, J. A. Sbarbaro, and R. R. Reves. "Short-term Incarceration for the Management of Noncompliance with Tuberculosis Treatment." *Chest* 112 (1997): 57-62; L. Singleton, M. Turner,

R. Haskal, S. Etkind, M. Tricano, and E. Nardell. "Long-term Hospitalization for Tuberculosis Control: Experience with a Medical-Psychosocial Inpatient Unit." *Journal of the American Medical Association* 278 (1997): 838-42.

28. W. J. Burman, D. L. Cohn, C. A. Rietmetjer, F. N. Judson, J. A. Sbarbara, and R. R. Reves. "Short-term Incarceration for the Management of Noncompliance with Tuberculosis Treatment." *Chest* 112 (1997) 57-62.

29. K. E. Thorpe. *Trends in the Distribution of Health Insurance Coverage Among New Yorkers, 1990-1996.* New York: United Hospital Fund, 1998.

30. *The Second Wave: The Looming Homeless Crisis in the Post-Entitlement Era.* New York: Coalition for the Homeless, 1996.

31. J. DeParle. "Success, and Frustration, as Welfare Rules Change." *New York Times,* December 30, 1997: Al, A16, A17.

32. A. Finder. "Welfare Clients Outnumber Jobs They Might Fill." *New York Times,* August 25, 1996: Al.

33. R. L. Swarns. "In Bronx Club, Welfare Mothers Prepare for Jobs, and Then Wait." *New York Times,* August 3l, 1997: Al.

34. DeParle, "Success, and Frustration, as Welfare Rules Change."

35. Ibid.

36. "Information Summary 1997."

37. M. D. Iseman and J. Starke. "Immigrants and Tuberculosis Control." *New England Journal of Medicine* 332 (1995): 1094-95.

38. U.S. Department of Commerce, Bureau of the Census.

39. S. Asch, L. Leake, R. Anderson, and L. Gelberg. "Why Do Symptomatic Patients Delay Obtaining Care for Tuberculosis?" *American Journal of Respiratory and Critical Care Medicine* 157 (1998): 1244-48.

40. I. Shapiro and R. Greenstein. *Trends in the Distribution of After-Tax Income.* Washington, DC: Center on Budget and Policy Priorities, 1997.

41. U.S. Department of Commerce, Bureau of the Census.

42. K. Larin and E. McNichol. "The Long-term Trend: The Late 1970s to the mid-1990s." *Pulling Apart: A State-by-State Analysis of Income Trends.* Washington, DC: Center on Budget and Policy Priorities, 1997.

43. S. Aaronson and S. V. Cameron. *Poverty in New York City, 1996: An Update and Perspectives.* New York: Community Service Society of New York, 1997.

44. P. Passell. "Benefits Dwindle Along with Wages for the Unskilled." *New York Times,* June 14, 1998: 1, 28.

45. Ibid.; J. DeParle, "In Booming Economy, Poor Still Struggle to Pay Rent." *New York Times,* June 16, 1998: A14.

46. U.S. Dept. of Commerce, Bureau of the Census.

47. Aaronson and Cameron, *Poverty in New York City.*

48. Ibid.

CHAPTER 6

1. New York City, N.Y., Health Code 11.47 (1993).

2. Response to Public Comments Concerning Proposed Amendments to Section 11.47 of Health Code. To: Hamburg, M.; From: Henning, K. New York: Department of Health, 1993.

3. R. Bayer, N. N. Dubler, and S. Landesman. "The Dual Epidemics of Tuberculosis and AIDS: Ethical and Policy Issues in Screening and Treatment." *American Journal of Public Health* 83 (1993): 649-54.

4. D. J. Rothman. "The Single Disease Hospital: Why Tuberculosis Justifies a Departure that AIDS Does Not." *Journal of Law, Medicine, and Ethics* 21, nos. 3-4 (1993): 296-302.

5. *School Board of Nassau County, Fl. v. Arline*, 480 U.S. 273, 288 (1987); L. O. Gostin. "Conference Proceedings: Public Health Powers: The Imminence of Radical Change. The Dual Epidemics of Tuberculosis and AIDS: Health Care Policy, Professional Practice, Law and Ethics." *New York City* (1992): 268-90.

6. H. D. Banta. "What Is Health Care?" In: A. R. Kovner, ed., *Health Care Delivery in the United States.* New York: Springer, 1990.

7. H. M. Leichter. *Free to Be Foolish: Politics and Health Promotion in the United States and Great Britain.* Princeton, NJ: Princeton University Press, 1991.

8. J. A. Sbarbaro. "Skin Testing in the Diagnosis of Tuberculosis." *Seminars in Respiratory Infections* 1 (1986): 234-38.

9. K. A. Sepkowitz. "How Contagious Is Tuberculosis?" *Clinical Infectious Diseases* 23 (1996): 954-62.

10. R. L. Riley, C. C. Mills, and F. O'Grady. "Infectiousness of Air from a Tuberculosis Ward—Ultraviolet Irradiation of Infected Air: Comparative Infectiousness of Different Patients." *American Review of Respiratory Disease* 84 (1962): 511-17; R. L. Riley, M. Knight, and G. Middlebrook. "Ultraviolet Susceptibility of BCG and Virulent *Tubercle* Bacilli." *American Review of Respiratory Disease* 113 (1976): 413-18.

11. L. Sultan, W. Nyka, C. Mills, F. O'Grady, W. Wells, and R. L. Riley. "Tuberculosis Disseminators. A Study of the Variability of Aerial Infectivity of Tuberculous Patients." *American Review of Respiratory Disease* 82 (1960): 358-69.

12. R. G. Loudon and S. K. Spohn. "Cough Frequency and Infectivity in Patients with Pulmonary Tuberculosis." *American Review of Respiratory Disease* 99 (1969): 109-11; F. M. McPhedran and E. L. Opie EL. "The Spread of Tuberculosis in Families." *American Journal of Hygiene* 22 (1935): 565-643; G. Hertzberg G. "The Infectiousness of Human Tuberculosis. *Acta Tuberculosea et Pneumologica Scandinavica* 38 (S-1) (1957): 1-146; J. B. Shaw and N. Wynn-Williams. "Infectivity of Pulmonary Tuberculosis in Relation to Sputum Status." Am Rev Tuberc 69 (1954): 724-32; R. G. Loudon, J. Williamson, and J. M. Johnson. "An Analysis of 3,485 Tuberculosis Contacts in the City of Edinburgh during 1954-1955." American Review of Tuberculosis 77 (1958): 623-43; H. A. van Guens, J. Meijer, and K. Styblo. "Results of Contact Examination in Rotterdam, 1967-1969." *Bulletin of the International Union Against Tuberculosis* 50 (1975): 107-21; S. Grzybowski, G. D. Barnett, and K. Styblo. "Contacts of Cases of Active Pulmonary Tuberculosis." *Bulletin of the International Union Against Tuberculosis* 50 (1975): 90-106.

13. McPhedran and Opie, "Spread of Tuberculosis in Families"; Hertzberg, "Infectiousness of Human Tuberculosis"; Shaw and Wynn-Williams, "Infectivity of Pulmonary Tuberculosis"; Loudon, Williamson, and Johnson,

"Analysis of 3,485 Tuberculosis Contacts"; van Guens, Meijer, and Styblo, "Results of Contact Examination in Rotterdam"; Grzybowski, Barnett, and Styblo, "Contacts of Cases of Active Pulmonary Tuberculosis."

14. K. Styblo. "Etat actuel de la question: epiderniologie de la tuberculose." *Bulletin of the International Union Against Tuberculosis* 53 (1978): 153-66.

15. J. Raffalli, K. A. Sepkowitz, and D. Armstrong. "Community Outbreaks of Tuberculosis: A Review." *Archives of Internal Medicine* 156 (1996): 1053-60.

16. S. E. Valway, M. P. Sanchez, T. F. Shinnick, et al. "An Outbreak Involving Extensive Transmission of a Virulent Strain of Mycobacterium Tuberculosis." *New England Journal of Medicine* 338 (1998): 633-39; S. M. Blower, P. M. Small, and P. C. Hopewell. "Control Strategies for Tuberculosis Epidemics: New Models for Old Problems." *Science* 273 (1996): 497-500.

17. Shaw and Wynn-Williams, "Infectivity of Pulmonary Tuberculosis"; Grzybowski, Barnett, and Styblo, "Contacts of Cases of Active Pulmonary Tuberculosis"; D. van Zwanenberg. "The Influence of the Number of Bacilli on the Development of Tuberculous Disease in Children." *American Review of Respiratory Disease* 82 (1960): 31-44.

18. A. Catanzaro. "Nosocomial Tuberculosis." *American Review of Respiratory Disease* 125 (1982): 559-62; G. Di Perri, M. Cruciam, M. C. Danzi, et al. "Nosocomial Epidemic of Active Tuberculosis among HIV-Infected Patients." *Lancet* 2 (1989): 1502-4.

19. R. Bellamy, C. Ruwende, T. Corrah, K. P. W. J. McAdam, H. C. Whittle, and A. V. S. Hill. "Variations in the NRAMPI Gene and Susceptibility to Tuberculosis in West Africans." *New England Journal of Medicine* 338 (1998): 640-44.

20. T. R. Frieden, L. F. Sherman, K. L. Maw, et al. "A Multi-institutional Outbreak of Highly Drug-Resistant Tuberculosis." *Journal of the American Medical Association* 276 (1996): 1229-35.

21. C. L. Daley, P. M. Small, G. F. Schecter, et al. "An Outbreak of Tuberculosis with Accelerated Progression among Persons Infected with the Human Immunodeficiency Syndrome." *New England Journal of Medicine* 326 (1992): 231-35; G. M. Cauthen, S. W. Dooley, I. M. Onorato, et al. "Transmission of Mycobacterium tuberculosis from Tuberculosis Patients with HIV Infection of AIDS." *American Journal of Epidemiology* 144 (1996): 169-77.

22. B. P. Vareldzis, J. Grosset, I. de Kantor, et al. "Drug-resistant Tuberculosis: Laboratory Issues. World Health Organization Recommendations." *Tubercule and Lung Disease* 75 (1994): 1-7.

23. A. Rouillon, S. Perdrizet, and R. Parrot. "Transmission of *Tubercle* Bacilli: The Effects of Chemotherapy." *Tubercle* 57 (1976): 275-99.

24. Singapore Tuberculosis Service/British Medical Research Council. "Clinical Trial of Three 6-month Regimens of Chemotherapy Given Intermittently in the Continuation Phase in the Treatment of Pulmonary Tuberculosis." *American Review of Respiratory Disease* 132 (1985): 374-78; Singapore Tuberculosis Service/British Medical Research Council. "Five-year Follow-up of a Clinical Trial of Three 6-month Regimens of Chemotherapy Given Intermittently in the Continuation Phase in the Treatment of Pulmonary Tuberculosis." *American Review of Respiratory Medicine* 137 (1988): 1147-50;

Singapore Tuberculosis Service/British Medical Research Council. "Assessment of a Daily Combined Preparation of Isomazid, Rifampin and Pyrazinamide in a Controlled Trial of Three 6-month Regimens for Smear-Positive Pulmonary Tuberculosis." *American Review of Respiratory Disease* 143 (1991): 707-12.

25. East African/British Medical Research Councils Study. "Controlled Clinical Trial of Five Short-Course (4-month) Chemotherapy Regimens in Pulmonary Tuberculosis—Second Report of the 4th Study." *American Review of Respiratory Disease* 123 (1981): 165; Hong Kong Chest Service/Tuberculosis Research Centre, Madras/British Medical Research Council. "A Controlled Trial of 2-month, 3-month, and 12-month Regimens of Chemotherapy for Sputum-Smear-Negative Pulmonary Tuberculosis. Results at 60 Months." *American Review of Respiratory Disease* 130 (1984): 23-28.

26. Sultan et al., "Tuberculosis Disseminators"; Loudon and Spohn, "Cough Frequency and Infectivity in Patients"; R. Newman, B. Doster, F. J. Murray, and S. F. Woolpert. "Rifampicin in Initial Treatment of Pulmonary Tuberculosis. A US Public Health Service Tuberculosis Therapy Trial." *American Review of Respiratory Disease* 103 (1971): 461-76.

27. S. E. Weis, P. C. Slocum, F. X. Blais, et al. "The Effect of Directly Observed Therapy on the Rates of Drug Resistance and Relapse in Tuberculosis." *New England Journal of Medicine* 330 (1994): 1179-84.

28. K. Brudney and J. Dobkin. "Resurgent Tuberculosis in New York City: Human Immunodeficiency Virus, Homelessness and the Decline of Tuberculosis Control Programmes." *American Review of Respiratory Disease* 144 (1991): 745-49.

29. E. L. Trudeau. "Environment in its Relation to the Progress of Bacterial Invasion in Tuberculosis." *Transactions of the American Climatological Association* 4, no. 13 (1887): 131-36.

30. R. H. Shyrock. *National Tuberculosis Association, 1904-1954: A Study of the Voluntary Health Movement in the United States.* New York: National Tuberculosis Association, 1957; M. M. Davis and M. C. Jarrett. *A Health Inventory of New York City.* New York: Welfare Council of New York City, 1929.

31. G. J. Drolet and A. M. Lowell. *A Half Century's Progress against Tuberculosis in New York City 1900-1950.* New York: New York Tuberculosis and Health Association, 1952; D. F. Musto. "Popular and Public Health Responses to Tuberculosis in America after 1870." In: V. A. Harden and G. B. Risse, eds. *AIDS and the Historian.* Washington, DC: U.S. Department of Health and Human Services, 1991.

32. T. McKeown. *The Role of Medicine: Dream, Mirage, or Nemesis?* Princeton, NJ: Princeton University Press, 1979.

33. J. Downes. "A Study of the Effectiveness of Certain Administrative Procedures in Tuberculosis Control." *Millbank Memorial Fund Quarterly* 14 (1936): 317-27.

34. A. L. Fairchild and G. M. Oppenheimer. "Public Health Nihilism versus Pragmatism: History, Politics, and the Control of Tuberculosis." *American Journal of Public Health* 88, no. 7 (1998): 1-14.

35. L. E. Holt. "A Report on One Thousand Tuberculin Tests in Young Children." *Proceedings of the Sixth International Congress on Tuberculosis* 2

(1908): 551-59.

36. A. K. Krause. *Rest and Other Things.* Baltimore: Williams & Wilkins, 1923.

37. L. G. Wilson. "The Historical Decline of Tuberculosis in Europe and America: Its Causes and Significance." *Journal of the History of Medicine and Allied Sciences* 45 (1990): 366-96.

38. Ibid.; L. G. Wilson. "The Rise and Fall of Tuberculosis in Minnesota: The Role of Infection." *Bulletin of the History of Medicine* 66 (1992): 16-52.

39. Fairchild and Oppenheimer, "Public Health Nihilism versus Pragmatism."

40. C. V. Ramakrishnan, R. H. Andrews, S. Devadatta, et al. "Influence of Segregation of Tuberculosis Patients for One Year on the Attack Rate of Tuberculosis in a 2-year Period in Close Family Contacts in South India." *Bulletin of the World Health Organization* 24 (1961): 129-48; S. R. Kamat, J. J. Y. Dawson, S. Devadatta, et al. "A Controlled Study of the Influence of Segregation of Tuberculous Patients for One Year on the Attack Rate of Tuberculosis in a 5-year Period in Close Family Contacts in South India." *Bulletin of the World Health Organization* 34 (1966): 517-32.

41. M. A. Behr, S. A. Warren, H. Salamon, et al. "Transmission of Mycobacterium tuberculosis from Patients Smear-Negative for Acid-Fast Bacilli." *Lancet* 353 (1999): 444-49.

42. Request to Amend Section 11.47 Health Code. From Kenneth Ong, Deputy Commissioner of Disease Intervention, to Margaret Hamburg, Commissioner of Health, New York City, October 6, 1992.

43. Brudney and Dobkin, "Resurgent Tuberculosis in New York City."

44. J. R. Newman. *The World of Mathematics: A Small Library of the Literature of Mathematics from A'h-Mose the Scribe to Albert Einstein.* Redmond, CA: Tempus Press, 1988.

45. D. Kahneman and A. Tversky. "The Psychology of Preferences." *Scientific American* 246 (1982): 160-73; D. Kahneman and A. Tversky. "Choices, Values, and Frames." *American Psychologist* 39 (1984): 341-50.

46. S. Lyall. "Scare or No, the Britons Are Still Mad about Beef." *New York Times,* January 26, 1998: A4.

47. J. Cocozza and H. J. Steadman. "The Failure of Psychiatric Predictions of Dangerousness: Clear and Convincing Evidence." *Rutgers Law Review* 29 (1976): 1084-101; H. J. Steadman. "Some Evidence on the Inadequacy of the Concept and Determination of Dangerousness in Law and Psychiatry." *Journal of Psychiatry and Law* 1 (1973): 409-26.

48. C. Hempel. "Valuation and Objectivity in Science." In: R. S. Cohen and L. Lauden, eds., *Physics, Philosophy and Psychoanalysis.* Boston: D. Reidel Publishing Co., 1983.

49. D. Kahneman and A. Tversky. "Subjective Probability." In: D. Kahneman, A. Tversky, and P. Slovic, eds. *Judgement under Uncertainty: Heuristics and Biases.* Cambridge: Cambridge University Press, 1981.

50. S. E. Valway, S. B. Richards, J. Kovacovich, R. B. Greifinger, J. T. Crawford, and S. W. Dooley. "Outbreak of Multi-Drug-Resistant Tuberculosis in a New York State Prison, 1991." *American Journal of Epidemiology* 140, no. 2 (1994): 113-22; C. Beck-Sague, S. W. Dooley, M. D. Hutton, et al. "Hospital Outbreak of Multidrug-Resistant Mycobacterium tuberculosis Infections— Factors in Transmission to Staff and HIV-infected Patients." *Journal of the*

American Medical Association 268 (1992): 1280-86; M. L. Pearson, J. A. Jereb, T. R. Frieden, et al. "Nosocomial Transmission of Multidrug-Resistant Mycobacterium tuberculosis: A Risk to Patients and Health Workers." *Annals of Internal Medicine* 117 (1992): 191-96; B. R. Edlin, J. I. Tokars, M. H. Grieco, et al. "An Outbreak of Multidrug-Resistant Tuberculosis among Hospitalized Patients with the Acquired Immunodeficiency Syndrome." *New England Journal of Medicine* 326 (1992): 1514-21.

51. P. Slovic. "Perception of Risk." *Science* 236 (1987): 280-85.

52. D. Broderick. "Judge: Add TB Ward to Rikers." *New York Post,* January 25, 1992: 8.

53. R. Bayer. "Coal, Lead, Asbestos, and HIV." *Journal of Metals* 35, no. 9 (1993): 897-901.

54. J. Helms. "The AIDS-infected Physician—Are Criminal Penalties Necessary to Protect the Public Health? Yes, Protect Innocent Victims." *American Bar Association Journal* 77 (1991): 46.

55. C. Hall. "Mentally Ill 'Not a Major Threat to Strangers.'" *Electronic Telegraph,* December 13, 1998.

56. New York City Tuberculosis Working Group. "Developing a System for Tuberculosis Prevention and Care in New York City." In: N. N. Dubler, R. Bayer, S. Landesman, and A. White, eds. *The Tuberculosis Revival: Individual Rights and Societal Obligations in a Time of AIDS.* New York: United Hospitals Fund, 1992.

57. "Safeguarding the City against TB." *New York Post,* February 25, 1992:20; "Can Society Protect Itself?" *New York Post,* September 5, 1992:12.

58. D. Vogel. *National Styles of Regulation: Environmental Policy in Great Britain and the United States.* Ithaca, NY: Cornell University Press, 1986.

59. B. Kaur and P. Bingham. "Compulsory Removal to and Detention in Hospital in the Case of Notifiable Disease: A Survey of Public Health Doctors." *Public Health* 107 (1993): 199-204.

60. R. J. Coker. "Uncertainty, Civil Liberties, Coercion, and Public Health." *British Medical Journal* 318 (1999): 1434-35.

61. Ibid.

62. K. H. Tiegen, B. Wibecke, and P. Slovic. "Societal Risks as Seen by a Norwegian Public." *Journal of Behavioural Decision Making* 111, no. 1 (1988): 111.

63. L. H. Glantz. "Risky Business: Setting Public Health Policy for HIV-infected Health Care Professionals." *Milbank Quarterly* 70, no. 1 (1992): 43-79.

64. Royal Society Study Group. *Risk Analysis, Perception and Management.* London: Royal Society, 1992.

65. P. Greenough. "Intimidation, Coercion and Resistance in the Final Stages of the South Asian Smallpox Eradication Campaign, 1973-1975." *Social Science and Medicine* 41, no. 5 (1995): 633-45.

66. K. Shrader-Frechette. "Scientific Method, Antifoundationalism, and Public Decisionmaking. *Risk—Issues in Health & Safety* 1, no. 23 (1990): 23-37.

67. P. Slovic, B. Fischhoff, and S. Lichtenstein. "Facts and Fears: Understanding Perceived Risk." In: R. C. Schwing and W. A. Albers, eds. *Societal Risk Assessment: How Safe Is Safe Enough?* New York: Plenum Press, 1980.

68. S. M. Stigler. *The History of Statistics: The Measurement of Uncertainty Before*

1900. Cambridge, MA: The Belknap Press of Harvard University Press, 1986.

CHAPTER 7

1. J. Tierney. "New York's Parallel Lives." *New York Times Magazine,* October 19, 1997: 51-53.
2. A. de Tocqueville. *Democracy in America,* 12th ed. New York: Harper Perennial, 1988.
3. L. Rainwater and W. L. Yancey. *The Moynihan Report and the Politics of Controversy.* Cambridge, MA: The MIT Press, 1967.
4. W. J. Wilson. *The Truly Disadvantaged: The Inner City, the Underclass, and Public Policy.* Chicago: University of Chicago Press, 1987; R. Nathan R. "Will the Underclass Always Be with Us?" *Society* 24 (March-April 1987): 57-62.
5. D. K. Shipler. *A Country of Strangers: Blacks and Whites in America.* New York: Alfred A. Knopf, 1997.
6. R. D. Putnam. "Bowling Alone: America's Declining Social Capital." *Journal of Democracy* 6, no. 1 (1995): 65-78.
7. R. Wuthnow. "Morality, Spirituality, and Democracy." *Society* 35, no. 3 (1998): 37-43.
8. R. Putnam. "Tuning In, Tuning Out: The Strange Disappearance of Social Capital in America." *Political Science and Politics* (December 1995): 664-83.
9. M. Brodie. *The Four Americas: Government and Social Policy Through the Eyes of America's Multi-Racial and Multi-Ethnic Society.* Menlo Park, NJ: *Washington Post*/Kaiser Family Foundation/Harvard University Survey Project, 1995; R. Morin and D. Balz. "Americans Losing Trust in Each Other and Institutions." *Washington Post,* January 28, 1996: Al, A6.
10. Morin and Balz, "Americans Losing Trust in Each Other and Institutions."
11. I. Kawachi, B. P. Kennedy, K. Lochner, D. Prothrow-Stith. "Social Capital, Income Inequality, and Mortality." *American Journal of Public Health* 87, no. 9 (1997): 1491-98.
12. Tocqueville, *Democracy in America.*
13. S. M. Lipset. *The First New Nation.* New York: Basic Books, 1963.
14. S. M. Lipset. *American Exceptionalism: A Double-edge Sword.* London: Norton Book News, 1996.
15. R. Dahrendorf. *Life Chances: Approaches to Social and Political Theory.* London: Weidenfeld and Nicolson, 1979.
16. D. Riesman. "Egocentrism." *Encounter* 55 (August-September 1980): 19-28.
17. Toqueville, *Democracy in America;* C. Taylor. *The Ethics of Authenticity.* Cambridge, MA: Harvard University Press, 1991; F. A. Hayek. *The Constitution of Liberty.* Chicago: University of Chicago Press, 1960; F. A. Hayek. *Studies in Philosophy, Politics and Economics.* London: Routledge & Kegan Paul, 1967.
18. Taylor, *Ethics of Authenticity.*
19. Hayek, *The Constitution of Liberty;* Hayek, *Studies in Philosophy, Politics and Economics.*
20. Toqueville, *Democracy in America.*
21. J. R. Kluegel and E. R. Smith. *Beliefs About Inequality: Americans' Views of*

What Is and What Ought to Be. New York: Aldine de Gruyter, 1986.

22. S. C. Fischer, M. Hout, M. S. Jankowski, S. R. Lucas, A. Swidler, and K. Voss K. *Inequality by Design: Cracking the Bell Curve Myth.* Princeton, NJ: Princeton University Press, 1996.

23. E. Burkett. "Don't Tread on My Tax Rate." *New York Times Magazine,* April 26, 1998: 42-45;

24. G. Wills. "The War between the States . . . and Washington." *New York Times Magazine,* July 5, 1998: 26-29.

25. D. Yankelovich. *American Values and Public Policy: How Reciprocity and Other Beliefs Are Reshaping American Politics.* Washington, DC: Democratic Leadership Council, 1992.

26. C. Leadbeater. *Civic Spirit: The Big Idea for a New Political Era.* London: Demos, 1997.

27. R. Samuelson. *The Good Life and Its Discontents.* New York: Times Books, 1995.

28. H. McClosky and J. Zaller. *The American Ethos.* Cambridge, MA: Harvard University Press,1984.

29. J. L. Hochschild. "Equal Opportunity and the Estranged Poor." In: W. J. Wilson, ed., *The Ghetto Underclass.* Newbury Park, CA: Sage Publications, 1989; D. P. McMurrer and I. V. Sawhill. *Getting Ahead: Economic and Social Mobility in America.* Washington, DC: The Urban Institute Press, 1998.

30. McMurrer and Sawhill, *Getting Ahead.*

31. H. Belz. "Affirmative Action and American Equality: A Constitutional Perspective." In: K. L. Grasso and C. R. Castillo, eds., *Liberty Under Law: American Constitutionalism, Yesterday, Today and Tomorrow.* Lanham, MD: University Press of America, 1998.

32. J. A. Morone. *The Democratic Wish: Popular Participation and the Limits of American Government,* 2nd ed. New Haven, CT: Yale University, 1998.

33. J. Rawls. *A Theory of Justice.* Cambridge, MA: Harvard University Press, 1971.

34. N. Daniels. "Health-care Needs and Distributive Justice." *Philosophy and Public Affairs* 10 (1981): 146-79.

35. G. Calabresi and P. Bobbitt. *Tragic Choices.* New York: W. W. Norton & Company, 1978.

36. Ibid.

37. "The Perception of Poverty in Europe." Commission of the European Community, 1977.

38. M. Kettle. "Americans Reluctant to Pay Their Dues." *Guardian Weekly,* April 19, 1998: 6.

39. J. R. Kluegel and M. Miyano. "Justice Beliefs and Support for the Welfare State in Advanced Capitalism." In: J. R. Kluegel, D. S. Mason, and B. Wegener, eds. *Social Justice and Political Change: Public Opinion in Capitalist and Post-Communist States.* New York: Aldine de Gruyter, 1995.

40. D. Rothman. "The State as Parent: Social Policy in the Progressive Era." In: W. Gaylin, I. Glasser, S. Marcus, and D. Rothman, eds. *Doing Good: The Limits of Benevolence.* New York: Pantheon Books, 1978.

41. I. Glasser. "Prisoners of Benevolence: Power versus Liberty in the Welfare State." In: W. Gaylin, I. Glasser, S. Marcus, and D. Rothman, eds. *Doing*

Good: The Limits of Benevolence. New York: Pantheon Books, 1978: 97-170.

42. Morin and Balz, "Americans Losing Trust in Each Other and Institutions."

43. Rothman, "The State as Parent."

44. T. Caplow. "Beyond Coca Cola: Europe and the American Way." *The Tocqueville Review* 18, no. 2 (1997): 157-61.

45. G. Vidal. "The State of the Union: 1975." *Esquire* (May 1975). Reprinted in: *United States—Essays, 1952-1992.* New York: Random House, 1993.

46. D. Rosner. "Health Care for the 'Truly Needy': Nineteenth-Century Origins of the Concept." *Milbank Memorial Fund Quarterly/Health and Society* 60, no. 3 (1982): 355-85.

47. P. Conrad and J. W. Schneider. *Deviance and Medicalization: From Badness to Sickness.* Philadelphia: Temple University Press, 1992.

48. W. Ryan. *Blaming the Victim.* New York: Vintage Books, 1971.

49. M. Ignatieff. *The Needs of Strangers: An Essay on Privacy, Solidarity, and the Politics of Being Human.* New York: Viking Penguin, 1986.

50. T. Lewin. "From Welfare Roll to Child Care Worker." *New York Times,* April 29, 1998: A14.

51. "Welfare Recipients Face Addiction Screening." *New York Times,* June 29, 1998: 136.

52. R. J. Samuelson. "Here's Some Good News, America." *Newsweek,* January 31, 1994: 43.

53. Wilson, *The Truly Disadvantaged;* C. Murray. *Losing Ground: American Social Policy, 1950-1980.* New York: Basic Books, 1984; L. Mead. *Beyond Entitlement: The Social Obligation of Citizenship.* New York: The Free Press, 1986; W. J. Wilson. *When Work Disappears: The World of the New Urban Poor.* New York: Alfred A. Knopf, 1996; S. Farkas. "Public Attitudes toward Welfare and Welfare Reform: A Focus Group Report by Public Agenda." Henry J. Kaiser Family Foundation, 1995.

54. D. Anderson, ed. *The Loss of Virtue: Moral Confusion & Social Disorder in Britain and America.* London: The Social Affairs Unit, 1992.

55. E. Goode. "Strange Bedfellows: Ideology, Politics, and Drug Legalization." *Society* 35, no. 4 (1998): 19-27.

56. R. Bayer. *Private Acts, Social Consequences: AIDS and the Politics of Public Health.* New York: The Free Press, 1989.

57. P. M. Boffey. "Reagan Urges Wide AIDS Testing But Does Not Call for Compulsion." *New York Times,* June 1, 1987: A1, A5.

58. M. Boyd. "President Urges Abstinence for Young to Avoid AIDS." *New York Times,* April 2, 1987: A10.

59. A. A. Skolnick. "'Collateral Casualties' Climb in Drug War." *Journal of the American Medical Association* 271, no. 21 (1994): 1636-39.

60. J. Mann. "Playing Politics with the Public's Health." *Washington Post,* April 29, 1998: D15.

61. K. S. Mitra. "Activists Claim NJ in Crisis State without Exchange." *Boston Globe,* January 12, 1999.

62. Centers for Disease Control. "HIV/AIDS Surveillance Report, 1997. Atlanta, Georgia." U.S. Department of Health and Human Services, Public Health Service, 9, no.2, 1997.

63. Skolnick, "'Collateral Casualties' Climb in Drug War."

64. Mann, "Playing Politics with the Public's Health."
65. E. Marines. "Busted: America's War on Marijuana." Public Broadcasting Service, Channel 13 (*Frontline*), 1998.
66. Editorial. "Judge Sweet's Beggars." *New York Post,* October 6, 1992:18.
67. P. W. Brickner, L. K. Scharer, B. A. Conanan, M. Savarese, and B. C. Scanlan, eds. *Under the Safety Net: The Health and Social Welfare of the Homeless in the United States.* New York: W. W. Norton & Co., 1992.
68. Editorial. "Homeless Families: Dinkins Comes Around. *New York Post,* September 8, 1992:18.
69. N. N. Bock, J. E. McGowan Jr., and H. M. Blumberg. "Few Opportunities Found for Tuberculosis Prevention among the Urban Poor." *International Journal of Tuberculosis and Lung Disease* 2, no. 2 (1998): 1249.
70. M. R Gasner, K. L. Maw, G. E. Feldman, P. I. Fujiwara, and T. R. Frieden. "The Use of Legal Action in New York City to Ensure Treatment of Tuberculosis." *New England Journal of Medicine* 340 (1998): 359-66.
71. L. B. Reichman. "The U-shaped Curve of Concern." *American Review of Respiratory Disease* 144 (1991): 741-42.
72. Morone, *The Democratic Wish.*
73. N. Glazer. *We Are All Multiculturalists Now.* Cambridge, MA: Harvard University Press, 1997.
74. Fischer et al., *Inequality by Design.*
75. R. J. Coker. "Lessons from New York's Tuberculosis Epidemic: Tuberculosis Is a Political as Much as a Medical Problem and So Are the Solutions." *British Medical Journal* 317 (1998): 616.

CHAPTER 8

1. D. Sassoon. Introduction. In: D. Sassoon, ed. *Looking Left: Socialism in Europe after the Cold War.* New York: The New Press, 1997.
2. I. Macwhirter. *Observer,* November 19, 1995.
3. A. Blair. "The Rights We Enjoy Reflect the Duties We Owe." The Spectator Lecture, 1995.
4. A. Blair. "The Flavour of Success." *Guardian,* July 6, 1995.
5. C. Leys. "The British Labour Party since 1989." In: D. Sassoon, ed. *Looking Left: Socialism in Europe after the Cold War.* New York: The New Press, 1997.
6. T. Ali. *Guardian,* October 28, 1996.
7. A. Pablos-Mendez, M. C. Raviglione, A. Laszlo, et al. "Global Surveillance for Antituberculosis-Drug Resistance, 1994-1997." *New England Journal of Medicine* 338 (1998): 1641-49.
8. L. P. Ormerod, A. Charlett, C. Gilliam, J. H. Darbyshire, and J. M. Watson. "Geographical Distribution of Tuberculosis in National Surveys of England and Wales in 1998 and 1993: Report of the Public Health Laboratory Service/ British Thoracic Society/Department of Health Collaborative Group. *Thorax* 53, no. 3 (1998): 176-81.
9. J. Newhouse. *Europe Adrift.* New York: Pantheon Books, 1997.
10. G. Young. "On a Journey through Borders of Hate." *Guardian Weekly,* June 28, 1998:24-25.
11. "Could Russia Go Fascist?" *The Economist,* July 11, 1998: 19-21.

12. Young, "On a Journey through Borders of Hate."

13. D. Williams. "Brutal Crimes of the Asylum Seekers." *Daily Mail,* November 30, 1998: 1, 4-5; M. Reynolds and A. Ramsay. "When 'Asylum' Means a Free Pass to Paradise." *Evening Standard,* October 15, 1998: 5.

14. W. Bagehot. *The English Constitution.* London: C. A. Watts & Co., 1964.

15. R. J. Coker. "Uncertainty, Civil Liberties, Coercion, and Public Health." *British Medical Journal* 318 (1999): 1434-35.

16. Ibid.; A. Hayward. *Tuberculosis Control in London: The Need for Change. A Report for The Thames Regional Directors of Public Health (A Discussion Document).* London: NHS Executive, 1998; A. Gordon. "TB Refugee 'Must Be Held in Hospital.'" *The Mail on Sunday,* August 30, 1998: 15.

17. Coker, "Uncertainty, Civil Liberties, Coercion, and Public Health"; P. Ormerod. "More Carrot or More Stick or Both?" *Thorax* 54 (1999): 96-97.

CHAPTER 9

18. "Estimates of Future Global Tuberculosis Morbidity and Mortality." *Morbidity and Mortality Weekly Report* 42, no. 49 (1993): 961-64.

19. A. Stone. *Regulation and Its Alternatives.* Washington, DC: Congressional Quarterly Press, 1982.

20. H. M. Leichter. *Free to Be Foolish: Politics and Health Promotion in the United States and Great Britain.* Princeton, NJ: Princeton University Press, 1991.

21. T. B. Macaulay. *Speeches.* London: Longman, Brown, Green and Longman's, 1854.

22. D. F. Musto. "Quarantine and the Problem of AIDS." *Milbank Quarterly* 64, Supplement 10 (1986): 97-117.

23. R. Bayer. *Private Acts, Social Consequences: AIDS and the Politics of Public Health.* New York: The Free Press, 1989.

24. Author interview with T. R. Frieden, June 29, 1998.

25. *Colyar v. Third Judicial District Court,* 469 F. Supp. 424 (D. Utah 1979).

26. Bayer, *Private Acts, Social Consequences.*

27. R. Steinbrook. "Battling HIV on Many Fronts." *New England Journal of Medicine* 37 (1997): 779-81; Council of State and Territorial Epidemiologists. *National HIV Surveillance: Addition to the National Public Health Surveillance System.* Atlanta: Council of State and Territorial Epidemiologists, 1997.

28. G. N. Colfax and A. B. Bindman. "Health Benefits and Risks of Reporting HIV-infected Individuals by Name." *American Journal of Public Health* 88 (1998): 876-79.

29. "Florida Investigates Breach of Confidentiality in HIV Records." *AIDS Policy Law* 11, no. 18 (1996): 1; P. A. Meyer, J. L. Jones, C. Z. Garrison, and H. Dowda. "Comparison of Individuals Receiving Anonymous and Confidential Testing for HIV." *Southern Medical Journal* 87 (1994): 344-47; E. J. Fordyce, S. Sambula, and R. Stoneburner. "Mandatory Reporting of Human Immunodeficiency Virus Testing Would Deter Blacks and Hispanics from Being Tested." *Journal of the American Medical Association* 262 (1989): 349.

30. R. Bellamy, C. Ruwende, T. Corrah, K. P. W. J. McAdam, H. C. Whittle, and A. V. S. Hill. "Variations in the NRAMP1 Gene and Susceptibility to

Tuberculosis in West Africans." *New England Journal of Medicine* 338 (1998): 640-44.

31. S. N. Tesh. *Hidden Arguments.* New Brunswick, NJ: Rutgers University Press, 1988.

32. M. A. Hamburg. "Public Health and Urban Medicine." *Lancet* 348 (1996): 1008-10.

33. C. McCord and H. P. Freeman. "Excess Mortality in Harlem." *New England Journal of Medicine* 322 (1990): 173-77.

34. A. Garfinkel. *The Ethics of Explanation.* New Haven, CT: Yale University Press, 1981.

35. L. Eisenberg, ed. *The Relevance of Social Sciences to Medicine.* Dordrecht: Reidel, 1981.

BIBLIOGRAPHY

Allport, F. "The J-curve Hypothesis of Conforming Behaviour." *Journal of Social Psychology* 5 (1934): 141-83.

Anderson, D,. ed. *The Loss of Virtue: Moral Confusion and Social Disorder in Britain and America.* London: The Social Affairs Unit, 1992.

Anderson, G. "In Search of Value: An International Comparison of Cost, Access, and Outcomes." *Health Affairs* 16, no. 6 (1997): 163-71.

Arno, P. S,. Murray, C. J. L,. Bonuck, K. A,. Alcabes, P. "The Economic Impact of Tuberculosis in Hospitals in New York City: A Preliminary Analysis." *Journal of Law, Medicine and Ethics* 21, no. 3-4 (1993): 317-23.

Ball, C. A,. and Barnes, M. "Public Health and Individual Rights: Tuberculosis Control and Detention Procedures in New York City." *Yale Law and Policy Review* 12, no. 1 (1994): 38-67.

Bayer, R. *Private Acts, Social Consequences: AIDS and the Politics of Public Health.* New York: The Free Press, 1989.

Brickner, P. W,. Scharer, L. K,. Conanan, B,. Elvy, A,. and Savarese, M,. eds. *Health Care of Homeless People.* New York: Springer, 1985.

Brickner, P. W,. Scharer, L. K,. Conanan, B. A,. Savarese, M,. and Scanlan, B. C,. eds. *Under the Safety Net: the Health and Social Welfare of the Homeless in the United States.* New York: W. W. Norton & Co,. 1992.

Brudney, K. "Homelessness and TB: A Study in Failure." *Journal of Law, Medicine and Ethics* 21, no. 3-4 (1993): 360-67.

Brudney, K,. and Dobkin, J. "Resurgent Tuberculosis in New York City: Human Immunodeficiency Virus, Homelessness and the Decline of Tuberculosis Control Programmes." *American Review of Respiratory Disease* 144 (1991): 745-49.

———. "A Tale of Two Cities: Tuberculosis Control in Managua and New York City." *Seminars in Respiratory Infections* 6 (1991): 261-72.

Bryder, L. *Below the Magic Mountain: A Social History of Tuberculosis in Twentieth-century Britain.* Oxford: Oxford University Press, 1988.

Calabresi, G,. and Bobbitt, P. *Tragic Choices.* New York: W. W. Norton & Co,. 1978.

Cassedy, J. H. Charles, V. *Chapin and the Public Health Movement.* Cambridge, MA: Harvard University Press, 1962.

Chapin, C. V. "History of State and Municipal Control of Disease." In: M. P. Ravenal, ed,. *A Half Century of Public Health.* New York: American Public Health Association, 1921, 135-37.

Davis, K,. and Rowland, D. "Financing Health Care for the Poor." In: E. Ginzberg, ed,. *Health Services Research: Key to Health Policy.* Cambridge, MA: Harvard University Press, 1991, 93-125.

Dennis, D. L,. and Monahan, J,. eds. *Coercion and Aggressive Community Treatment: A New Frontier in Mental Health Law.* New York: Plenum Press, 1996.

Donziger, S. R,. ed. *The Real War on Crime.* New York: Harper, 1996.

Dormandy, T. *The White Death: A History of Tuberculosis.* London: The Hambledon Press, 1999.

Drolet, G. J,. and Lowell, A. M. *A Half Century's Progress against Tuberculosis in New York City, 1900-1950.* New York: New York Tuberculosis and Health Association, 1952.

Eisenberg, L,. ed. *The Relevance of Social Sciences to Medicine.* Dordrecht: Reidel, 1981

Ellwood, D. T. *Poor Support: Poverty in the American family.* New York: Basic Books, 1988.

Fairchild, A. L,. and Oppenheimer, G. M. "Public Health Nihilism versus Pragmatism: History, Politics, and the Control of Tuberculosis." *American Journal of Public Health* 88 (1988): 1-14.

Farley, R,. ed. *State of the Union: America in the 1990s.* New York: Russell Sage Foundation, 1995.

Feldberg, G. D. *Disease and Class: Tuberculosis and the Shaping of Modern North American Society.* New Brunswick, NJ: Rutgers University Press.

Fischer, S. C,. Hout, M,. Jankowski, M. S,. Lucas, S. R,. Swidler, A,. and Voss, K. *Inequality by Design: Cracking the Bell Curve Myth.* Princeton, NJ: Princeton University Press, 1996.

Fishkin, J. *Justice, Equal Opportunity and the Family.* New Haven, CT: Yale University Press, 1983.

Foreman, C. H,. Jr. *Plagues, Products & Politics: Emergent Public Health Hazards and National Policymaking.* Washington, DC: The Brookings Institution, 1994.

Frankl, V. E. *Man's Search for Meaning.* 4th ed. Boston: Beacon Press, 1992.

Frieden, T. R,. Fujiwara, P. I,. Washko, R. M,. and Hamburg, M. A. "Tuberculosis in New York City—Turning the Tide." *New England Journal of Medicine* 333 (1995): 229-33.

Frieden, T. R,. Sherman, L. F,. Maw, K. L,. et al. "A Multi-Institutional Outbreak of Highly Drug-Resistant Tuberculosis." *Journal of the American Medical Association* 276 (1996): 1229-35.

Frieden, T. R,. Sterling, T,. Pablos-Mendez, A,. Kilburn, J. O,. Cauthen, G. M,. and Dooley, S. W. "The Emergence of Drug-resistant Tuberculosis in New York City." *New England Journal of Medicine* 328 (1993): 521-26.

Frieden, T. R,. Woodley, C. L,. Crawford, J. T,. Lew, D,.and Dooley, S. M. "The Molecular Epidemiology of Tuberculosis in New York City: The Importance of Nosocomial Transmission and Laboratory Error." *Tubercle and Lung Disease* 77 (1996): 407-13.

Gasner, M. R,. Maw, K. L,. Feldman, G. E,. Fujiwara, P. I,. and Frieden, T. R. "The Use of Legal Action in New York City to Ensure Treatment of Tuberculosis." *New England Journal of Medicine* 340 (1998): 359-66.

Gaylin, W,. and Jennings, B. *The Perversion of Autonomy: The Proper Uses of Coercion and Constraints in a Liberal Society.* New York: The Free Press, 1996.

Glazer, N. *We Are All Multiculturalists Now.* Cambridge, MA: Harvard University Press, 1997.

Gostin, L. O. "Controlling the Resurgent Tuberculosis Epidemic: A 50-state Survey of TB Statutes and Proposals for Reform." *Journal of the American Medical Association* 269 (1993): 255-61.

———. "The Resurgent Tuberculosis Epidemic in the Era of AIDS: Reflections on Public Health, Law, and Society." *Maryland Law Review* 54, no. 1 (1995): 1-131.

Gottschalk, P,. and Smeeding, T. M. "Cross-national Comparisons of Earnings and Income Inequality." *Journal of Economic Literature* 35 (1997): 633-87.

Grad, F. P. *The Public Health Law Manual,* 2nd ed. Washington, DC: American Public Health Association, 1990.

Ignatieff, M. *The Needs of Strangers: An essay on Privacy, Solidarity, and the Politics of Being Human.* New York: Viking Penguin, 1986.

Jencks, C. *Rethinking Social Policy: Race, Poverty, and the Underclass.* Cambridge, MA: Harvard University Press, 1992.

Jencks, C,. and Peterson, P. E,. eds. *The Urban Underclass.* Washington, DC: The Brookings Institution, 1991.

Johnstone, J. W. C. "Social Class, Social Areas and Delinquency." *Sociology and Social Research* 63 (1978): 49-72.

Kahneman, D,. and Tversky, A. "Choices, Values, and Frames." *American Psychologist* 39 (1984): 341-50.

———. "The Psychology of Preferences." *Scientific American* 246 (1982): 160-73.

Kahneman, D,. and Tversky, A. "Subjective Probability." In: D. Kahneman, A. Tversky, and P. Slovic, eds,. *Judgement under Uncertainty: Heuristics and Biases.* Cambridge: Cambridge University Press, 1981.

Katz, M. B. *In the Shadow of the Poorhouse: A Social History of Welfare in America.* New York: Basic Books, 1986.

———. *The Undeserving Poor: From the War on Poverty to the War on Welfare.* New York: Pantheon Books, 1989.

Kerckhoff, A. C,. ed. *Generations and the Lifecourse.* Boulder, CO: Westview Press, 1995.

Knopf, S. A. *Tuberculosis as a Disease of the Masses and How to Combat It,* 4th ed. New York: Fred P. Flori, 1907.

La Fond, J. Q,. and Durham, M. L. *Back to the Asylum: The Future of Mental Health Law and Policy in the United States.* New York: Oxford University Press, 1992.

Leichter, H. M. *Free to be Foolish: Politics and Health Promotion in the United States and Great Britain.* Princeton, NJ: Princeton University Press, 1991.

Lerner, B. H. "'On What Authority Is This Being Done?' Tuberculosis Control, Poverty and Coercion in Seattle, 1909-1973." Ph.D. diss,. University of Washington, Seattle, 1996.

Lipset, S. M. *American Exceptionalism: A Double-edge Sword.* London: Norton Book News, 1996.

———. *The First New Nation.* New York: Basic Books, 1963.

Mayho, P. *The Tuberculosis Survival Handbook.* London: XLR8, 1999.

McAdams, D. P. *The Person: An Introduction to Personality Psychology.* London: Harcourt Brace Jovanovich, 1990.

McCord, C,. and Freeman, H. P. "Excess Mortality in Harlem." *New England Journal of Medicine* 322 (1990): 173-77.

McKeown, T. *The Role of Medicine: Dream, Mirage, or Nemesis?* Princeton, NJ: Princeton University Press, 1979.

McMurrer, D. P,. and Sawhill, I. V. *Getting Ahead: Economic and Social Mobility in America.* Washington, DC: The Urban Institute Press, 1998.

Morone, J. A. *The Democratic Wish: Popular Participation and the Limits of American Government,* 2nd ed. New Haven, CT: Yale University Press, 1998.

Newhouse, J. *Europe Adrift.* New York: Pantheon Books, 1997.

Palmer, J. L,. and Sawhill, I. V,. eds. *The Reagan Experiment.* Washington, DC: Urban Institute Press, 1982.

Peterson, P,. ed. *The New Urban Reality.* Washington, DC: The Brookings Institution, 1985.

Porter, D,. ed. *The History of Public Health and the Modern State.* Amsterdam: Rodopi BV, 1994.

Porter, D,. Porter, R. "The Enforcement of Health: The British Debate." In: E. Fee and D. M. Fox, eds,. *AIDS: The Burdens of History.* Berkeley: University of California Press, 1988, 97-120.

Putnam, R. D. "Bowling Alone: America's Declining Social Capital." *Journal of Democracy* 6, no. 1 (1995): 65-78.

———. "Tuning In, Tuning Out: The Strange Disappearance of Social Capital in America." *Political Science and Politics,* December (1995): 664-83.

Rawls, J. *A Theory of Justice.* Cambridge, MA: Harvard University Press, 1971.

Reinarman, C,. and Levine, H. G,. eds. *Crack in America: Demon Drugs and Social Justice.* Berkeley: University of California Press, 1997.

Rhoden, N. "The Limits of Liberty: Deinstitutionalization, Homelessness, and Libertarian Theory." *Emory Law Journal* 31, no. 2 (1982): 375-440.

Rosner, D. "Health Care for the 'Truly Needy': Nineteenth-century Origins of the Concept." *Milbank Memorial Fund Quarterly/Health and Society* 60, no. 3 (1982): 355-85.

Rossi, P. H. *Down and Out in America: The Origins of Homelessness.* Chicago: University of Chicago Press, 1989.

Rothman, D. J. "The Single Disease Hospital: Why Tuberculosis Justifies a Departure That AIDS Does Not." *Journal of Law, Medicine and Ethics* 21, nos. 3-4 (1993): 296-302.

Rothman, S. M. *Living in the Shadow of Death: Tuberculosis and the Social Experience of Illness in American History.* Baltimore: Johns Hopkins University Press, 1995.

———. "Seek and Hide: Public Health Departments and Persons with Tuberculosis, 1890-1940." *Journal of Law, Medicine and Ethics* 21, nos. 3-4 (1993): 289-95.

Ryan, F. *Tuberculosis: The Greatest Story Never Told.* Bromsgrove, England: Swift Publishers, 1992.

Sassoon, D,. ed. *Looking Left: Socialism in Europe after the Cold War.* New York: The New Press, 1997.

Schaffer, D. R. *Social and Personality Development,* 3rd ed. Pacific Grove, CA: Brooks/Cole Publishing Company, 1994.

Schwing, R. C,. and Albers, W. A,. eds. *Societal Risk Assessment: How Safe is Safe Enough?* New York: Plenum Press, 1980.

Sepkowitz, K. A,. Telzak, E. E,. Recalde, S,. and Armstrong, D. "Trends in Susceptibility of Tuberculosis in New York City, 1987-1991." *Clinical Infectious Diseases* 18 (1994): 755-59.

Shipler, D. K. *A Country of Strangers: Blacks and Whites in America.* New York: Alfred A. Knopf, 1997.

Starr, P. *The Social Transformation of American Medicine.* New York: Basic Books, 1982.

Sumartojo, E. "When Tuberculosis Treatment Fails: A Social Behavioural Account of Patient Adherence." *American Review of Respiratory Disease* 147 (1993): 1311-20.

Taylor, C. *The Ethics of Authenticity.* Cambridge, MA: Harvard University Press, 1991.

Tesh, S. N. *Hidden Arguments.* New Brunswick, NJ: Rutgers University Press, 1988.

Tilly, C. *Durable Inequalities*. Berkeley: University of California Press, 1998.

Tocqueville, A. de. *Democracy in America*, 12th ed. New York: Harper Perennial, 1988.

Trudeau, E. L. "Environment in Its Relation to the Progress of Bacterial Invasion in Tuberculosis." *Transactions of the American Climatological Association* 4 (1887): 131-36.

The Tuberculosis Revival: Individual Rights and Societal Obligations in a Time of AIDS. New York: United Hospital Fund, 1992.

Valway, S. E,. Greifinger, R. B,. Papania, M,. et al. "Multidrug-resistant Tuberculosis in the New York State Prison System, 1990-1991." *Journal of Infectious Diseases* 170 (1994): 151-56.

Wallace, D. "Roots of Increased Health Care Inequality in New York." *Society, Science and Medicine* 31, no. 11 (1990): 1219-27.

Wallace, R. "Contagion and Incubation in New York City Structural Fires, 1964-76." *Human Ecology* 6, no. 4 (1978): 423-33.

————. "Fire Service Productivity and the New York City Fire Crisis: 1968-1979." *Human Ecology* 9, no. 4 (1981): 433-64.

Wallace, R,. and Wallace, D. "Origins of Public Health Collapse in New York City: The Dynamics of Planned Shrinkage, Contagious Urban Decay and Social Disintegration." *Bulletin of the New York Academy of Medicine* 66, no. 5 (1990): 391-434.

Wilson, W. J. *The Truly Disadvantaged: The Inner City, the Underclass, and Public Policy*. Chicago: University of Chicago Press, 1987.

————. *When Work Disappears: The World of the New Urban Poor*. New York: Alfred A. Knopf, 1996.

————, ed. *The Ghetto Underclass*. Newbury Park, CA: Sage Publications, 1993.

Winslow, C.-E. A. *The Life of Hermann Biggs*. Philadelphia: Lea and Febiger, 1929.

Yankelovich, D. *American Values and Public Policy: How Reciprocity and Other Beliefs Are Reshaping American Politics*. Washington, DC: Democratic Leadership Council, 1992.

Yoshikawa, H. "Long-term Effects of Early Childhood Programs on Social Outcomes and Delinquency." *The Future of Children* 5 (Winter 1995): 51-75

————. "Prevention as Cumulative Protection: Effects of Early Family Support and Education on Chronic Delinquency and Its Risks." *Psychological Bulletin* 115, no. 1 (1994): 28-54.

INDEX